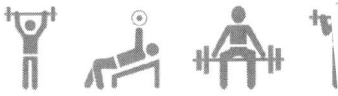

Gym Workout Log Book

Daily workout, meals and sleep tracker for a fitter and healthier you!

Copyright © 2018 Fit-For-Life Notebooks

All rights reserved.

ISBN: 1720404151
ISBN-13: 9781720404156

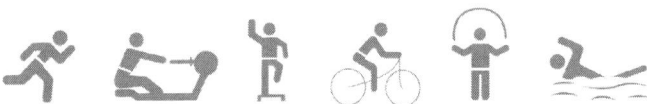

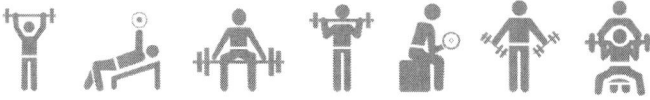

Name:

Contact:

_____

*"Patience, Persistence and Perspiration make an Unbeatable
Combination for Success"*

- Napoleon Hill

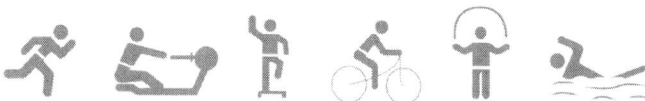

CONTENTS   PAGES

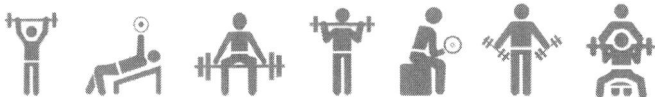

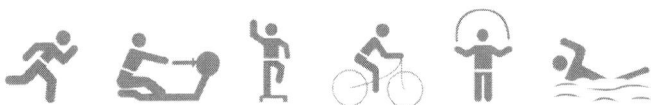

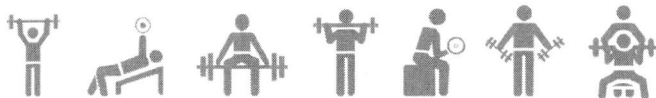

Daily Records

Today is a great day to train!

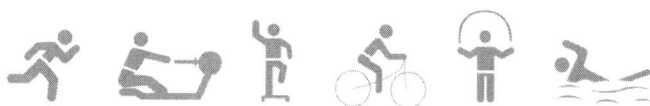

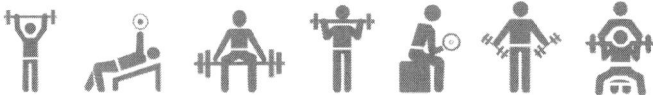

Day/Date: Mon, Jul 2   **Time/Duration:** 9am, 50 mins

WEIGHT TRAINING

Muscle Group(s) **Chest** **Shoulders** **Back** **Arms** **Legs** **Abs**

EXERCISE	Set 1 Weight	Set 1 Reps	Set 2 Weight	Set 2 Reps	Set 3 Weight	Set 3 Reps	Set 4 Weight	Set 4 Reps	Rest between Sets	Set 5 or the Set with Max. Wt./Reps Weight	Reps
Bench press	70	10	90	8	100	6	100	5	2	100	5
Bench press	100	5	90	6	80	5					
Inc dumbell press	40	10	50	7	60	6	70	4	2	70	4
Dumbell flys	20	10	25	8	25	8	30	5	1	3	5

Use two rows to note down exercises for which you do more than 5 sets.

Use this column to note your best set, or as set 5.

EXAMPLE

CARDIO & STRETCHING   **Time/Duration:** 4pm, 50 mins   *NOTES*

EXERCISE / LEVEL	Time/ Duration Goal	Time/ Duration Actual	Distance Goal	Distance Actual	Calories Goal	Calories Actual
Running	30	27	6	5	400	350
Rowing	20	20	4	4	150	150

Ideas/goals for next session:
Try increasing bench press weight by 10. Do more exercises for triceps.

DIET & SLEEP

MEALS	Protein	Carbs	Total Fat	Sugars	Sodium/ Salt	Fiber	Calories
BREAKFAST: Corn flakes, sandwich	15	☐				☐	700
LUNCH: Chicken caesar salad	25					☐	600
DINNER: Lasagna, bread	10	☐				☐	450
SNACKS: Cheese sandwich, croissant	8	☐				☐	600
DRINKS: Coffee (2), orange juice	2						150
TOTAL	60						2500

WATER (8-oz glasses OR 2 litres of water a day): 9   Yes ✕ No ✕

TOTAL SLEEP / REST HOURS	NIGHT	DAY	TOTAL
	7	1	8

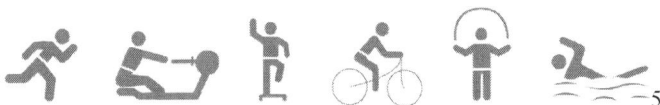

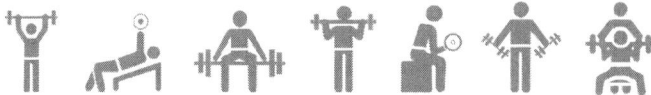

Day/Date:	Time/Duration:

WEIGHT TRAINING

Muscle Group(s)	Chest	Shoulders	Back	Arms	Legs	Abs

	Set 1		Set 2		Set 3		Set 4		Rest between Sets	Set 5 or the Set with Max. Wt./Reps	
EXERCISE	Weight	Reps	Weight	Reps	Weight	Reps	Weight	Reps		Weight	Reps

CARDIO & STRETCHING   Time/Duration: NOTES

EXERCISE / LEVEL	Time/ Duration		Distance		Calories		Ideas/goals for next session:
	Goal	Actual	Goal	Actual	Goal	Actual	

DIET & SLEEP

MEALS	Protein	Carbs	Total Fat	Sugars	Sodium/ Salt	Fiber	Calories
BREAKFAST:							
LUNCH:							
DINNER:							
SNACKS:							
DRINKS:							
TOTAL							

WATER (8-oz glasses OR 2 litres of water a day):		Yes	✕	No	✕

TOTAL SLEEP / REST HOURS	NIGHT	DAY	TOTAL

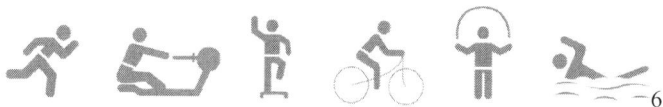

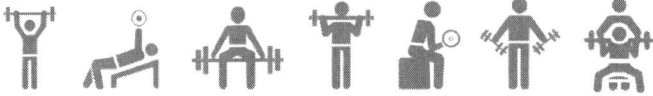

WEIGHT TRAINING

Day/Date: Time/Duration:

Muscle Group(s)	Chest	Shoulders		Back		Arms		Rest between Sets	Legs	Abs
	Set 1		Set 2		Set 3		Set 4		Set 5 or the Set with Max. Wt./Reps	
EXERCISE	Weight	Reps	Weight	Reps	Weight	Reps	Weight	Reps		Weight	Reps

CARDIO & STRETCHING

Time/Duration: NOTES

EXERCISE / LEVEL	Time/Duration		Distance		Calories		Ideas/goals for next session:
	Goal	Actual	Goal	Actual	Goal	Actual	

DIET & SLEEP

MEALS	Protein	Carbs	Total Fat	Sugars	Sodium/Salt	Fiber	Calories
BREAKFAST:							
LUNCH:							
DINNER:							
SNACKS:							
DRINKS:							
TOTAL							

WATER (8-oz glasses OR 2 litres of water a day):   Yes   x   No   x

TOTAL SLEEP / REST HOURS	NIGHT	DAY	TOTAL

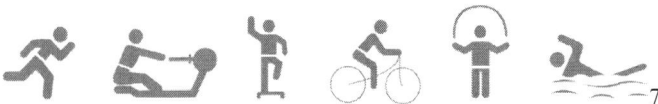

7

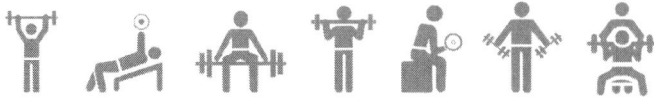

WEIGHT TRAINING

Day/Date: Time/Duration:

Muscle Group(s)   Chest   Shoulders   Back   Arms   Legs   Abs

EXERCISE	Set 1 Weight	Set 1 Reps	Set 2 Weight	Set 2 Reps	Set 3 Weight	Set 3 Reps	Set 4 Weight	Set 4 Reps	Rest between Sets	Set 5 or the Set with Max. Wt./Reps Weight	Reps

CARDIO & STRETCHING   Time/Duration: NOTES

EXERCISE / LEVEL	Time/Duration Goal	Actual	Distance Goal	Actual	Calories Goal	Actual

Ideas/goals for next session:

DIET & SLEEP

MEALS	Protein	Carbs	Total Fat	Sugars	Sodium/ Salt	Fiber	Calories
BREAKFAST:							
LUNCH:							
DINNER:							
SNACKS:							
DRINKS:							
TOTAL							

WATER (8-oz glasses OR 2 litres of water a day):	Yes	X	No	X

TOTAL SLEEP / REST HOURS	NIGHT	DAY	TOTAL

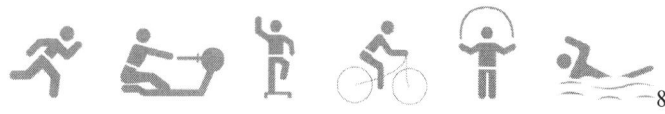

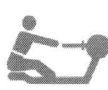

Day/Date: **Time/Duration:**

WEIGHT TRAINING

Muscle Group(s)	Chest		Shoulders		Back		Arms		Rest between Sets	Set 5 or the Set with Max. Wt./Reps	
	Set 1		Set 2		Set 3		Set 4				
EXERCISE	Weight	Reps	Weight	Reps	Weight	Reps	Weight	Reps		Weight	Reps

CARDIO & STRETCHING   Time/Duration: NOTES

EXERCISE / LEVEL	Time/Duration		Distance		Calories		Ideas/goals for next session:
	Goal	Actual	Goal	Actual	Goal	Actual	

DIET & SLEEP

MEALS	Protein	Carbs	Total Fat	Sugars	Sodium/ Salt	Fiber	Calories
BREAKFAST:							
LUNCH:							
DINNER:							
SNACKS:							
DRINKS:							
TOTAL							

WATER (8-oz glasses OR 2 litres of water a day):		Yes ✕	No ✕
TOTAL SLEEP / REST HOURS	NIGHT	DAY	TOTAL

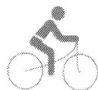
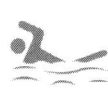

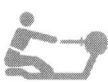

WEIGHT TRAINING

Day/Date: Time/Duration:

Muscle Group(s)	Chest		Shoulders		Back		Arms		Rest between Sets	Legs Abs Set 5 or the Set with Max. Wt./Reps	
	Set 1		Set 2		Set 3		Set 4				
EXERCISE	Weight	Reps	Weight	Reps	Weight	Reps	Weight	Reps		Weight	Reps

CARDIO & STRETCHING   Time/Duration:

NOTES

Ideas/goals for next session:

EXERCISE / LEVEL	Time/Duration		Distance		Calories	
	Goal	Actual	Goal	Actual	Goal	Actual

DIET & SLEEP

MEALS	Protein	Carbs	Total Fat	Sugars	Sodium/Salt	Fiber	Calories
BREAKFAST:							
LUNCH:							
DINNER:							
SNACKS:							
DRINKS:							
TOTAL							

WATER (8-oz glasses OR 2 litres of water a day):		Yes	×	No	×

TOTAL SLEEP / REST HOURS	NIGHT	DAY	TOTAL

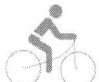
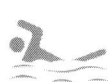

10

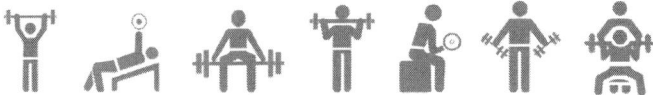

Day/Date: _____   **Time/Duration:** _____

WEIGHT TRAINING

Muscle Group(s)   Chest   Shoulders   Back   Arms   Legs   Abs

EXERCISE	Set 1 Weight	Set 1 Reps	Set 2 Weight	Set 2 Reps	Set 3 Weight	Set 3 Reps	Set 4 Weight	Set 4 Reps	Rest between Sets	Set 5 or the Set with Max. Wt./Reps Weight	Reps

CARDIO & STRETCHING   Time/Duration: _____   NOTES

Ideas/goals for next session:

EXERCISE / LEVEL	Time/Duration Goal	Actual	Distance Goal	Actual	Calories Goal	Actual

DIET & SLEEP

MEALS	Protein	Carbs	Total Fat	Sugars	Sodium/Salt	Fiber	Calories
BREAKFAST:							
LUNCH:							
DINNER:							
SNACKS:							
DRINKS:							
TOTAL							

WATER (8-oz glasses OR 2 litres of water a day):		Yes	×	No	×

TOTAL SLEEP / REST HOURS	NIGHT	DAY	TOTAL

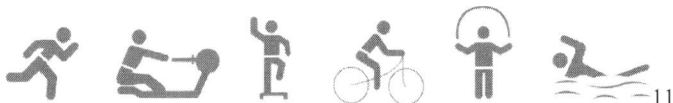

WEIGHT TRAINING

Day/Date: Time/Duration:

Muscle Group(s)	Chest		Shoulders		Back		Arms		Rest between Sets	Legs Abs Set 5 or the Set with Max. Wt./Reps	
EXERCISE	Set 1		Set 2		Set 3		Set 4				
	Weight	Reps	Weight	Reps	Weight	Reps	Weight	Reps		Weight	Reps

CARDIO & STRETCHING   Time/Duration: *NOTES*

EXERCISE / LEVEL	Time/ Duration		Distance		Calories		Ideas/goals for next session:
	Goal	Actual	Goal	Actual	Goal	Actual	

DIET & SLEEP

MEALS	Protein	Carbs	Total Fat	Sugars	Sodium/ Salt	Fiber	Calories
BREAKFAST:							
LUNCH:							
DINNER:							
SNACKS:							
DRINKS:							
TOTAL							

WATER (8-oz glasses OR 2 litres of water a day):		Yes	✕	No	✕

TOTAL SLEEP / REST HOURS	NIGHT	DAY	TOTAL

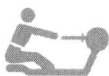 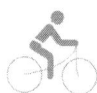

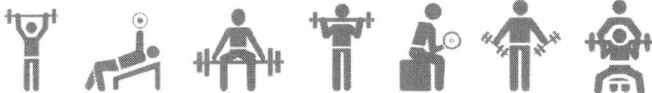

WEIGHT TRAINING

Day/Date: Time/Duration:

Muscle Group(s)	Chest		Shoulders		Back		Arms		Rest between Sets	Legs Abs — Set 5 or the Set with Max. Wt./Reps	
	Set 1		Set 2		Set 3		Set 4				
EXERCISE	Weight	Reps	Weight	Reps	Weight	Reps	Weight	Reps		Weight	Reps

CARDIO & STRETCHING

Time/Duration: NOTES

Ideas/goals for next session:

EXERCISE / LEVEL	Time/Duration		Distance		Calories	
	Goal	Actual	Goal	Actual	Goal	Actual

DIET & SLEEP

MEALS	Protein	Carbs	Total Fat	Sugars	Sodium/ Salt	Fiber	Calories
BREAKFAST:							
LUNCH:							
DINNER:							
SNACKS:							
DRINKS:							
TOTAL							

WATER (8-oz glasses OR 2 litres of water a day):		Yes ✕	No ✕
TOTAL SLEEP / REST HOURS	**NIGHT**	**DAY**	**TOTAL**

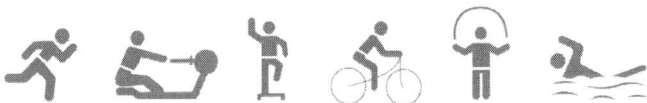

13

Day/Date: *Time/Duration:*

WEIGHT TRAINING

| *Muscle Group(s)* | Chest | | Shoulders | | Back | | Arms | | Rest between Sets | Legs | Abs |
| | Set 1 | | Set 2 | | Set 3 | | Set 4 | | | Set 5 or the Set with Max. Wt./Reps | |
EXERCISE	Weight	Reps	Weight	Reps	Weight	Reps	Weight	Reps		Weight	Reps

CARDIO & STRETCHING   Time/Duration: NOTES

| EXERCISE / LEVEL | Time/ Duration | | Distance | | Calories | | Ideas/goals for next session: |
	Goal	Actual	Goal	Actual	Goal	Actual	

DIET & SLEEP

MEALS	Protein	Carbs	Total Fat	Sugars	Sodium/ Salt	Fiber	Calories
BREAKFAST:							
LUNCH:							
DINNER:							
SNACKS:							
DRINKS:							
TOTAL							

WATER (8-oz glasses OR 2 litres of water a day):		Yes ✕	No ✕
TOTAL SLEEP / REST HOURS	NIGHT	DAY	TOTAL

Day/Date: **Time/Duration:**

WEIGHT TRAINING

Muscle Group(s)   Chest   Shoulders   Back   Arms   Legs   Abs

EXERCISE	Set 1 Weight	Set 1 Reps	Set 2 Weight	Set 2 Reps	Set 3 Weight	Set 3 Reps	Set 4 Weight	Set 4 Reps	Rest between Sets	Set 5 or the Set with Max. Wt./Reps Weight	Reps

CARDIO & STRETCHING   Time/Duration: NOTES

Ideas/goals for next session:

EXERCISE / LEVEL	Time/Duration Goal	Actual	Distance Goal	Actual	Calories Goal	Actual

DIET & SLEEP

MEALS	Protein	Carbs	Total Fat	Sugars	Sodium/Salt	Fiber	Calories
BREAKFAST:							
LUNCH:							
DINNER:							
SNACKS:							
DRINKS:							
TOTAL							

WATER (8-oz glasses OR 2 litres of water a day):   Yes   ✕   No   ✕

TOTAL SLEEP / REST HOURS	NIGHT	DAY	TOTAL

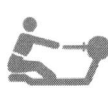 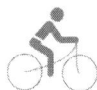 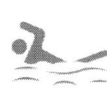

WEIGHT TRAINING

Day/Date: Time/Duration:

Muscle Group(s)	Chest		Shoulders		Back		Arms		Rest between Sets	Legs	Abs
	Set 1		Set 2		Set 3		Set 4			Set 5 or the Set with Max. Wt./Reps	
EXERCISE	Weight	Reps	Weight	Reps	Weight	Reps	Weight	Reps		Weight	Reps

CARDIO & STRETCHING

Time/Duration: NOTES

EXERCISE / LEVEL	Time/ Duration		Distance		Calories		Ideas/goals for next session:
	Goal	Actual	Goal	Actual	Goal	Actual	

DIET & SLEEP

MEALS	Protein	Carbs	Total Fat	Sugars	Sodium/ Salt	Fiber	Calories
BREAKFAST:							
LUNCH:							
DINNER:							
SNACKS:							
DRINKS:							
TOTAL							

WATER (8-oz glasses OR 2 litres of water a day):		Yes ✕	No ✕
TOTAL SLEEP / REST HOURS	NIGHT	DAY	TOTAL

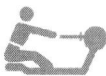

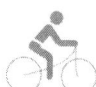

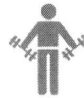

Day/Date: *Time/Duration:*

WEIGHT TRAINING

Muscle Group(s)   Chest   Shoulders   Back   Arms   Legs   Abs

EXERCISE	Set 1		Set 2		Set 3		Set 4		Rest between Sets	Set 5 or the Set with Max. Wt./Reps	
	Weight	Reps	Weight	Reps	Weight	Reps	Weight	Reps		Weight	Reps

CARDIO & STRETCHING   Time/Duration: NOTES

EXERCISE / LEVEL	Time/ Duration		Distance		Calories		Ideas/goals for next session:
	Goal	Actual	Goal	Actual	Goal	Actual	

DIET & SLEEP

MEALS	Protein	Carbs	Total Fat	Sugars	Sodium/ Salt	Fiber	Calories
BREAKFAST:							
LUNCH:							
DINNER:							
SNACKS:							
DRINKS:							
TOTAL							

WATER (8-oz glasses OR 2 litres of water a day):	Yes ✕ No ✕		
TOTAL SLEEP / REST HOURS	**NIGHT**	**DAY**	**TOTAL**

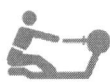

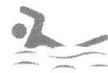

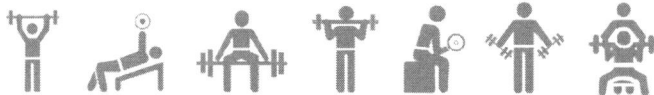

Day/Date: **Time/Duration:**

WEIGHT TRAINING

Muscle Group(s)   Chest   Shoulders   Back   Arms   Legs   Abs

EXERCISE	Set 1		Set 2		Set 3		Set 4		Rest between Sets	Set 5 or the Set with Max. Wt./Reps	
	Weight	Reps	Weight	Reps	Weight	Reps	Weight	Reps		Weight	Reps

CARDIO & STRETCHING   Time/Duration: NOTES

EXERCISE / LEVEL	Time/ Duration		Distance		Calories		Ideas/goals for next session:
	Goal	Actual	Goal	Actual	Goal	Actual	

DIET & SLEEP

MEALS	Protein	Carbs	Total Fat	Sugars	Sodium/ Salt	Fiber	Calories
BREAKFAST:							
LUNCH:							
DINNER:							
SNACKS:							
DRINKS:							
TOTAL							

WATER (8-oz glasses OR 2 litres of water a day):   Yes   ✕   No   ✕

TOTAL SLEEP / REST HOURS	NIGHT	DAY	TOTAL

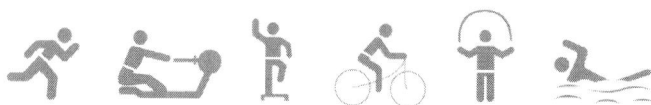

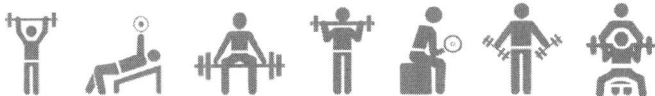

Day/Date: _____   Time/Duration: _____

WEIGHT TRAINING

Muscle Group(s)   Chest   Shoulders   Back   Arms   Legs   Abs

EXERCISE	Set 1 Weight	Set 1 Reps	Set 2 Weight	Set 2 Reps	Set 3 Weight	Set 3 Reps	Set 4 Weight	Set 4 Reps	Rest between Sets	Set 5 or the Set with Max. Wt./Reps Weight	Reps

CARDIO & STRETCHING   Time/Duration: _____   NOTES

EXERCISE / LEVEL	Time/Duration Goal	Actual	Distance Goal	Actual	Calories Goal	Actual	Ideas/goals for next session:

DIET & SLEEP

MEALS	Protein	Carbs	Total Fat	Sugars	Sodium/Salt	Fiber	Calories
BREAKFAST:							
LUNCH:							
DINNER:							
SNACKS:							
DRINKS:							
TOTAL							

WATER (8-oz glasses OR 2 litres of water a day):	Yes ☒	No ☒

TOTAL SLEEP / REST HOURS	NIGHT	DAY	TOTAL

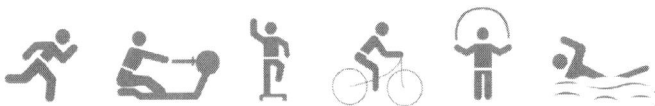

19

WEIGHT TRAINING

Day/Date: Time/Duration:

Muscle Group(s)	Chest		Shoulders		Back		Arms		Rest between Sets	Legs / Abs Set 5 or the Set with Max. Wt./Reps	
	Set 1		Set 2		Set 3		Set 4				
EXERCISE	Weight	Reps	Weight	Reps	Weight	Reps	Weight	Reps		Weight	Reps

CARDIO & STRETCHING   Time/Duration: NOTES

EXERCISE / LEVEL	Time/ Duration		Distance		Calories		Ideas/goals for next session:
	Goal	Actual	Goal	Actual	Goal	Actual	

DIET & SLEEP

MEALS	Protein	Carbs	Total Fat	Sugars	Sodium/ Salt	Fiber	Calories
BREAKFAST:							
LUNCH:							
DINNER:							
SNACKS:							
DRINKS:							
TOTAL							

WATER (8-oz glasses OR 2 litres of water a day):		Yes ✕	No ✕
TOTAL SLEEP / REST HOURS	NIGHT	DAY	TOTAL

20

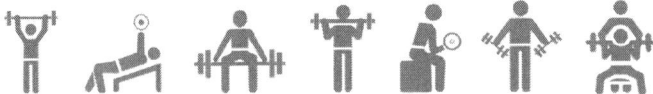

WEIGHT TRAINING

Day/Date: Time/Duration:

Muscle Group(s)	Chest		Shoulders		Back		Arms		Rest between Sets	Legs	Abs
	Set 1		Set 2		Set 3		Set 4			Set 5 or the Set with Max. Wt./Reps	
EXERCISE	Weight	Reps	Weight	Reps	Weight	Reps	Weight	Reps		Weight	Reps

CARDIO & STRETCHING

Time/Duration: NOTES

EXERCISE / LEVEL	Time/ Duration		Distance		Calories	
	Goal	Actual	Goal	Actual	Goal	Actual

Ideas/goals for next session:

DIET & SLEEP

MEALS	Protein	Carbs	Total Fat	Sugars	Sodium/ Salt	Fiber	Calories
BREAKFAST:							
LUNCH:							
DINNER:							
SNACKS:							
DRINKS:							
TOTAL							

WATER (8-oz glasses OR 2 litres of water a day):		Yes ✕	No ✕
TOTAL SLEEP / REST HOURS	**NIGHT**	**DAY**	**TOTAL**

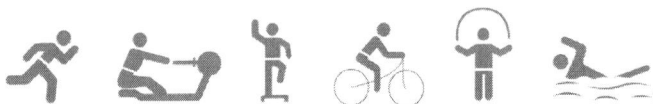

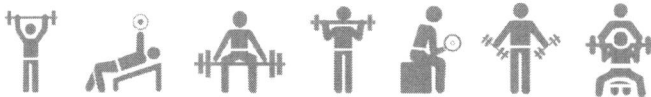

WEIGHT TRAINING

Muscle Group(s)	Chest		Shoulders		Back		Arms		Rest between Sets	Set 5 or the Set with Max. Wt./Reps	
	Set 1		Set 2		Set 3		Set 4				
EXERCISE	Weight	Reps	Weight	Reps	Weight	Reps	Weight	Reps		Weight	Reps

CARDIO & STRETCHING   Time/Duration: NOTES

EXERCISE / LEVEL	Time/ Duration		Distance		Calories		Ideas/goals for next session:
	Goal	Actual	Goal	Actual	Goal	Actual	

DIET & SLEEP

MEALS	Protein	Carbs	Total Fat	Sugars	Sodium/ Salt	Fiber	Calories
BREAKFAST:							
LUNCH:							
DINNER:							
SNACKS:							
DRINKS:							
TOTAL							

WATER (8-oz glasses OR 2 litres of water a day):   Yes   ✕   No   ✕

TOTAL SLEEP / REST HOURS	NIGHT	DAY	TOTAL

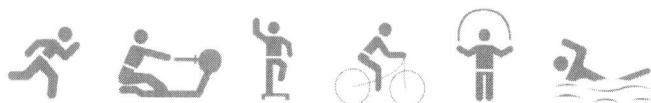

WEIGHT TRAINING

Day/Date: _____ Time/Duration: _____

Muscle Group(s)	Chest		Shoulders		Back		Arms			Legs	Abs
	Set 1		Set 2		Set 3		Set 4		Rest between Sets	Set 5 or the Set with Max. Wt./Reps	
EXERCISE	Weight	Reps	Weight	Reps	Weight	Reps	Weight	Reps		Weight	Reps

CARDIO & STRETCHING Time/Duration: _____ NOTES

EXERCISE / LEVEL	Time/ Duration		Distance		Calories		Ideas/goals for next session:
	Goal	Actual	Goal	Actual	Goal	Actual	

DIET & SLEEP

MEALS	Protein	Carbs	Total Fat	Sugars	Sodium/ Salt	Fiber	Calories
BREAKFAST:							
LUNCH:							
DINNER:							
SNACKS:							
DRINKS:							
TOTAL							
WATER (8-oz glasses OR 2 litres of water a day):			Yes ✕		No ✕		

TOTAL SLEEP / REST HOURS	NIGHT	DAY	TOTAL

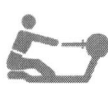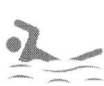

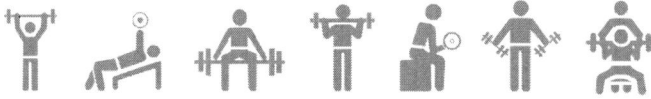

WEIGHT TRAINING

Day/Date: Time/Duration:

Muscle Group(s)	Chest		Shoulders		Back		Arms		Rest between Sets	Legs	Abs
	Set 1		Set 2		Set 3		Set 4			Set 5 or the Set with Max. Wt./Reps	
EXERCISE	Weight	Reps	Weight	Reps	Weight	Reps	Weight	Reps		Weight	Reps

CARDIO & STRETCHING   Time/Duration: NOTES

EXERCISE / LEVEL	Time/Duration		Distance		Calories		Ideas/goals for next session:
	Goal	Actual	Goal	Actual	Goal	Actual	

DIET & SLEEP

MEALS	Protein	Carbs	Total Fat	Sugars	Sodium/Salt	Fiber	Calories
BREAKFAST:							
LUNCH:							
DINNER:							
SNACKS:							
DRINKS:							
TOTAL							

WATER (8-oz glasses OR 2 litres of water a day):   Yes   ✕   No   ✕

TOTAL SLEEP / REST HOURS	NIGHT	DAY	TOTAL

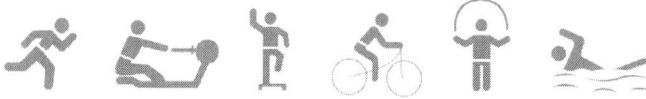

24

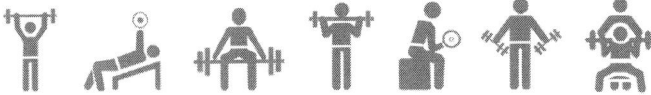

WEIGHT TRAINING

Day/Date: Time/Duration:

Muscle Group(s)   Chest   Shoulders   Back   Arms   Legs   Abs

EXERCISE	Set 1 Weight	Set 1 Reps	Set 2 Weight	Set 2 Reps	Set 3 Weight	Set 3 Reps	Set 4 Weight	Set 4 Reps	Rest between Sets	Set 5 or the Set with Max. Wt./Reps Weight	Reps

CARDIO & STRETCHING   Time/Duration: NOTES

Ideas/goals for next session:

EXERCISE / LEVEL	Time/ Duration Goal	Actual	Distance Goal	Actual	Calories Goal	Actual

DIET & SLEEP

MEALS	Protein	Carbs	Total Fat	Sugars	Sodium/ Salt	Fiber	Calories
BREAKFAST:							
LUNCH:							
DINNER:							
SNACKS:							
DRINKS:							
TOTAL							
WATER (8-oz glasses OR 2 litres of water a day):				Yes No			
TOTAL SLEEP / REST HOURS				NIGHT	DAY	TOTAL	

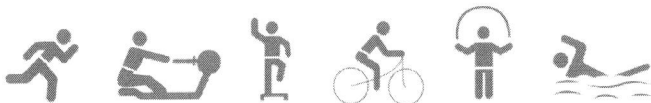

WEIGHT TRAINING

Day/Date: Time/Duration:

Muscle Group(s)	Chest		Shoulders		Back		Arms		Rest between Sets	Legs Abs Set 5 or the Set with Max. Wt./Reps	
	Set 1		Set 2		Set 3		Set 4				
EXERCISE	Weight	Reps	Weight	Reps	Weight	Reps	Weight	Reps		Weight	Reps

CARDIO & STRETCHING   Time/Duration: NOTES

EXERCISE / LEVEL	Time/ Duration		Distance		Calories		Ideas/goals for next session:
	Goal	Actual	Goal	Actual	Goal	Actual	

DIET & SLEEP

MEALS	Protein	Carbs	Total Fat	Sugars	Sodium/ Salt	Fiber	Calories
BREAKFAST:							
LUNCH:							
DINNER:							
SNACKS:							
DRINKS:							
TOTAL							

WATER (8-oz glasses OR 2 litres of water a day):   Yes   ✕   No   ✕

TOTAL SLEEP / REST HOURS	NIGHT	DAY	TOTAL

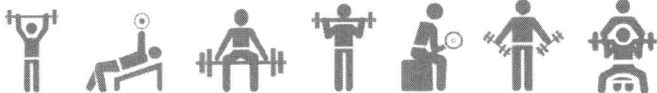

WEIGHT TRAINING

Day/Date: Time/Duration:

Muscle Group(s)   Chest   Shoulders   Back   Arms   Legs   Abs

EXERCISE	Set 1		Set 2		Set 3		Set 4		Rest between Sets	Set 5 or the Set with Max. Wt./Reps	
	Weight	Reps	Weight	Reps	Weight	Reps	Weight	Reps		Weight	Reps

CARDIO & STRETCHING   Time/Duration: NOTES

Ideas/goals for next session:

EXERCISE / LEVEL	Time/ Duration		Distance		Calories	
	Goal	Actual	Goal	Actual	Goal	Actual

DIET & SLEEP

MEALS	Protein	Carbs	Total Fat	Sugars	Sodium/ Salt	Fiber	Calories
BREAKFAST:							
LUNCH:							
DINNER:							
SNACKS:							
DRINKS:							
TOTAL							

WATER (8-oz glasses OR 2 litres of water a day):   Yes   ☒   No   ☒

TOTAL SLEEP / REST HOURS	NIGHT	DAY	TOTAL

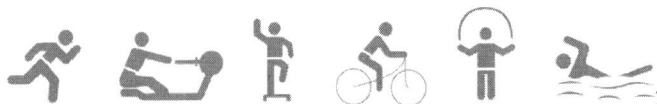

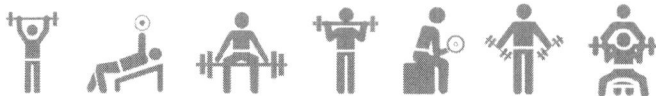

Day/Date: Time/Duration:

WEIGHT TRAINING

Muscle Group(s)	Chest		Shoulders		Back		Arms		Rest between Sets	Legs	Abs
	Set 1		Set 2		Set 3		Set 4			Set 5 or the Set with Max. Wt./Reps	
EXERCISE	Weight	Reps	Weight	Reps	Weight	Reps	Weight	Reps		Weight	Reps

CARDIO & STRETCHING   Time/Duration: NOTES

EXERCISE / LEVEL	Time/ Duration		Distance		Calories		Ideas/goals for next session:
	Goal	Actual	Goal	Actual	Goal	Actual	

DIET & SLEEP

MEALS	Protein	Carbs	Total Fat	Sugars	Sodium/ Salt	Fiber	Calories
BREAKFAST:							
LUNCH:							
DINNER:							
SNACKS:							
DRINKS:							
TOTAL							

WATER (8-oz glasses OR 2 litres of water a day):		Yes ✕ No ✕	
TOTAL SLEEP / REST HOURS	NIGHT	DAY	TOTAL

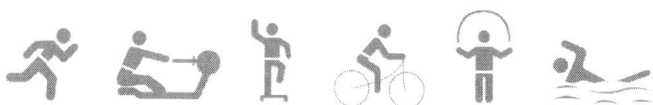

Day/Date: **Time/Duration:**

WEIGHT TRAINING

Muscle Group(s)	Chest		Shoulders		Back		Arms		Rest between Sets	Legs	Abs
	Set 1		Set 2		Set 3		Set 4			Set 5 or the Set with Max. Wt./Reps	
EXERCISE	Weight	Reps	Weight	Reps	Weight	Reps	Weight	Reps		Weight	Reps

CARDIO & STRETCHING   Time/Duration: NOTES

EXERCISE / LEVEL	Time/Duration		Distance		Calories		Ideas/goals for next session:
	Goal	Actual	Goal	Actual	Goal	Actual	

DIET & SLEEP

MEALS	Protein	Carbs	Total Fat	Sugars	Sodium/ Salt	Fiber	Calories
BREAKFAST:							
LUNCH:							
DINNER:							
SNACKS:							
DRINKS:							
TOTAL							

WATER (8-oz glasses OR 2 litres of water a day):		Yes ☒	No ☒

TOTAL SLEEP / REST HOURS	NIGHT	DAY	TOTAL

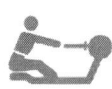 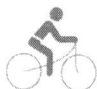 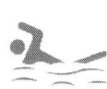

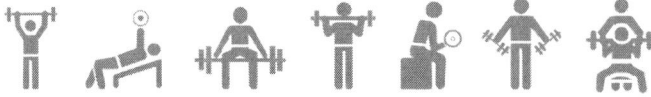

Day/Date: _____   Time/Duration: _____

WEIGHT TRAINING

Muscle Group(s)	Chest		Shoulders		Back		Arms		Rest between Sets	Legs Abs Set 5 or the Set with Max. Wt./Reps	
	Set 1		Set 2		Set 3		Set 4				
EXERCISE	Weight	Reps	Weight	Reps	Weight	Reps	Weight	Reps		Weight	Reps

CARDIO & STRETCHING   Time/Duration: _____   NOTES

EXERCISE / LEVEL	Time/ Duration		Distance		Calories		Ideas/goals for next session:
	Goal	Actual	Goal	Actual	Goal	Actual	

DIET & SLEEP

MEALS	Protein	Carbs	Total Fat	Sugars	Sodium/ Salt	Fiber	Calories
BREAKFAST:							
LUNCH:							
DINNER:							
SNACKS:							
DRINKS:							
TOTAL							

WATER (8-oz glasses OR 2 litres of water a day):		Yes ✕	No ✕
TOTAL SLEEP / REST HOURS	NIGHT	DAY	TOTAL

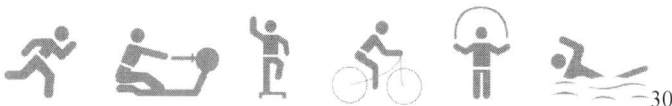

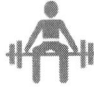

Day/Date: _____   Time/Duration: _____

WEIGHT TRAINING

Muscle Group(s)	Chest		Shoulders		Back		Arms		Rest between Sets	Legs Abs	
	Set 1		Set 2		Set 3		Set 4			Set 5 or the Set with Max. Wt./Reps	
EXERCISE	Weight	Reps	Weight	Reps	Weight	Reps	Weight	Reps		Weight	Reps

CARDIO & STRETCHING   Time/Duration: _____   NOTES

EXERCISE / LEVEL	Time/ Duration		Distance		Calories		Ideas/goals for next session:
	Goal	Actual	Goal	Actual	Goal	Actual	

DIET & SLEEP

MEALS	Protein	Carbs	Total Fat	Sugars	Sodium/Salt	Fiber	Calories
BREAKFAST:							
LUNCH:							
DINNER:							
SNACKS:							
DRINKS:							
TOTAL							

WATER (8-oz glasses OR 2 litres of water a day):	Yes	✕	No	✕

TOTAL SLEEP / REST HOURS	NIGHT	DAY	TOTAL

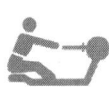 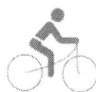 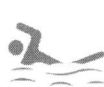

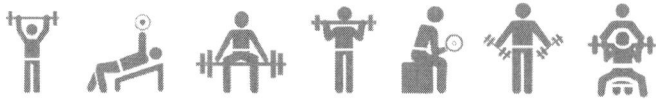

Day/Date: _____   **Time/Duration:** _____

WEIGHT TRAINING

Muscle Group(s)   **Chest**   **Shoulders**   **Back**   **Arms**   **Legs**   **Abs**

EXERCISE	Set 1 Weight	Set 1 Reps	Set 2 Weight	Set 2 Reps	Set 3 Weight	Set 3 Reps	Set 4 Weight	Set 4 Reps	Rest between Sets	Set 5 or the Set with Max. Wt./Reps Weight	Reps

CARDIO & STRETCHING   Time/Duration: _____   NOTES

Ideas/goals for next session:

EXERCISE / LEVEL	Time/ Duration Goal	Actual	Distance Goal	Actual	Calories Goal	Actual

DIET & SLEEP

MEALS	Protein	Carbs	Total Fat	Sugars	Sodium/ Salt	Fiber	Calories
BREAKFAST:							
LUNCH:							
DINNER:							
SNACKS:							
DRINKS:							
TOTAL							

WATER (8-oz glasses OR 2 litres of water a day):	Yes ☒	No ☒

TOTAL SLEEP / REST HOURS	NIGHT	DAY	TOTAL

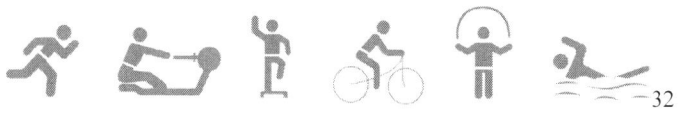

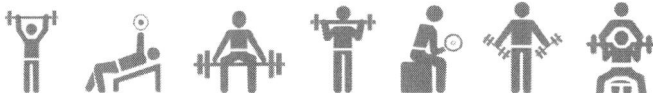

Day/Date: Time/Duration:

WEIGHT TRAINING

Muscle Group(s)	Chest	Shoulders	Back	Arms	Legs	Abs

EXERCISE	Set 1		Set 2		Set 3		Set 4		Rest between Sets	Set 5 or the Set with Max. Wt./Reps	
	Weight	Reps	Weight	Reps	Weight	Reps	Weight	Reps		Weight	Reps

CARDIO & STRETCHING   Time/Duration: NOTES

Ideas/goals for next session:

EXERCISE / LEVEL	Time/Duration		Distance		Calories	
	Goal	Actual	Goal	Actual	Goal	Actual

DIET & SLEEP

MEALS	Protein	Carbs	Total Fat	Sugars	Sodium/Salt	Fiber	Calories
BREAKFAST:							
LUNCH:							
DINNER:							
SNACKS:							
DRINKS:							
TOTAL							

WATER (8-oz glasses OR 2 litres of water a day):		Yes ✕	No ✕

TOTAL SLEEP / REST HOURS	NIGHT	DAY	TOTAL

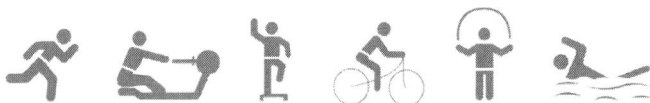

33

Day/Date: Time/Duration:

WEIGHT TRAINING

Muscle Group(s)   Chest   Shoulders   Back   Arms   Legs   Abs

| EXERCISE | Set 1 | | Set 2 | | Set 3 | | Set 4 | | Rest between Sets | Set 5 or the Set with Max. Wt./Reps | |
	Weight	Reps	Weight	Reps	Weight	Reps	Weight	Reps		Weight	Reps

CARDIO & STRETCHING   Time/Duration: NOTES

| EXERCISE / LEVEL | Time/Duration | | Distance | | Calories | | Ideas/goals for next session: |
	Goal	Actual	Goal	Actual	Goal	Actual	

DIET & SLEEP

MEALS	Protein	Carbs	Total Fat	Sugars	Sodium/ Salt	Fiber	Calories
BREAKFAST:							
LUNCH:							
DINNER:							
SNACKS:							
DRINKS:							
TOTAL							

WATER (8-oz glasses OR 2 litres of water a day):   Yes   ×   No   ×

TOTAL SLEEP / REST HOURS	NIGHT	DAY	TOTAL

34

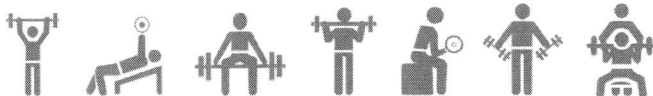

Day/Date: Time/Duration:

WEIGHT TRAINING

Muscle Group(s)   **Chest**   **Shoulders**   **Back**   **Arms**   **Legs**   **Abs**

EXERCISE	Set 1 Weight	Set 1 Reps	Set 2 Weight	Set 2 Reps	Set 3 Weight	Set 3 Reps	Set 4 Weight	Set 4 Reps	Rest between Sets	Set 5 or the Set with Max. Wt./Reps Weight	Reps

CARDIO & STRETCHING   Time/Duration: NOTES

EXERCISE / LEVEL	Time/Duration Goal	Actual	Distance Goal	Actual	Calories Goal	Actual	Ideas/goals for next session:

DIET & SLEEP

MEALS	Protein	Carbs	Total Fat	Sugars	Sodium/Salt	Fiber	Calories
BREAKFAST:							
LUNCH:							
DINNER:							
SNACKS:							
DRINKS:							
TOTAL							

WATER (8-oz glasses OR 2 litres of water a day):		Yes ✕	No ✕

TOTAL SLEEP / REST HOURS	NIGHT	DAY	TOTAL

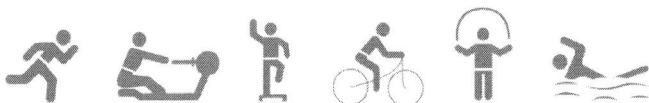

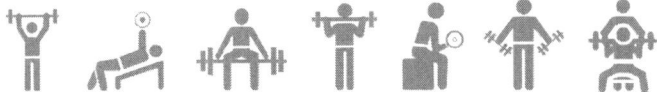

WEIGHT TRAINING

Day/Date: Time/Duration:

Muscle Group(s)	Chest		Shoulders		Back		Arms			Legs	Abs
	Set 1		Set 2		Set 3		Set 4		Rest between Sets	Set 5 or the Set with Max. Wt./Reps	
EXERCISE	Weight	Reps	Weight	Reps	Weight	Reps	Weight	Reps		Weight	Reps

CARDIO & STRETCHING

Time/Duration: NOTES

EXERCISE / LEVEL	Time/ Duration		Distance		Calories		Ideas/goals for next session:
	Goal	Actual	Goal	Actual	Goal	Actual	

DIET & SLEEP

MEALS	Protein	Carbs	Total Fat	Sugars	Sodium/ Salt	Fiber	Calories
BREAKFAST:							
LUNCH:							
DINNER:							
SNACKS:							
DRINKS:							
TOTAL							

WATER (8-oz glasses OR 2 litres of water a day):		Yes ✕	No ✕
TOTAL SLEEP / REST HOURS	NIGHT	DAY	TOTAL

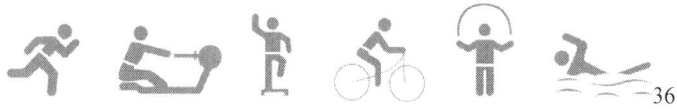

36

WEIGHT TRAINING

Day/Date: _____ Time/Duration: _____

Muscle Group(s)	Chest		Shoulders		Back		Arms		Rest between Sets	Legs	Abs
	Set 1		Set 2		Set 3		Set 4			Set 5 or the Set with Max. Wt./Reps	
EXERCISE	Weight	Reps	Weight	Reps	Weight	Reps	Weight	Reps		Weight	Reps

CARDIO & STRETCHING

Time/Duration: _____ NOTES

Ideas/goals for next session:

EXERCISE / LEVEL	Time/ Duration		Distance		Calories	
	Goal	Actual	Goal	Actual	Goal	Actual

DIET & SLEEP

MEALS	Protein	Carbs	Total Fat	Sugars	Sodium/ Salt	Fiber	Calories
BREAKFAST:							
LUNCH:							
DINNER:							
SNACKS:							
DRINKS:							
TOTAL							

WATER (8-oz glasses OR 2 litres of water a day):   Yes ×   No ×

TOTAL SLEEP / REST HOURS	NIGHT	DAY	TOTAL

Day/Date: _____   Time/Duration: _____

WEIGHT TRAINING

Muscle Group(s) **Chest**   **Shoulders**   **Back**   **Arms**   **Legs   Abs**

EXERCISE	Set 1 Weight	Set 1 Reps	Set 2 Weight	Set 2 Reps	Set 3 Weight	Set 3 Reps	Set 4 Weight	Set 4 Reps	Rest between Sets	Set 5 or the Set with Max. Wt./Reps Weight	Set 5 or the Set with Max. Wt./Reps Reps

CARDIO & STRETCHING   Time/Duration: _____   NOTES

EXERCISE / LEVEL	Time/Duration Goal	Time/Duration Actual	Distance Goal	Distance Actual	Calories Goal	Calories Actual

Ideas/goals for next session:

DIET & SLEEP

MEALS	Protein	Carbs	Total Fat	Sugars	Sodium/ Salt	Fiber	Calories
BREAKFAST:							
LUNCH:							
DINNER:							
SNACKS:							
DRINKS:							
TOTAL							

WATER (8-oz glasses OR 2 litres of water a day):   Yes ✕   No ✕

TOTAL SLEEP / REST HOURS	NIGHT	DAY	TOTAL

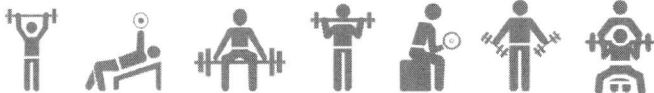

WEIGHT TRAINING

Day/Date: Time/Duration:

Muscle Group(s)   Chest   Shoulders   Back   Arms   Legs   Abs

EXERCISE	Set 1 Weight	Set 1 Reps	Set 2 Weight	Set 2 Reps	Set 3 Weight	Set 3 Reps	Set 4 Weight	Set 4 Reps	Rest between Sets	Set 5 or the Set with Max. Wt./Reps Weight	Reps

CARDIO & STRETCHING

Time/Duration: NOTES

Ideas/goals for next session:

EXERCISE / LEVEL	Time/ Duration Goal	Actual	Distance Goal	Actual	Calories Goal	Actual

DIET & SLEEP

MEALS	Protein	Carbs	Total Fat	Sugars	Sodium/ Salt	Fiber	Calories
BREAKFAST:							
LUNCH:							
DINNER:							
SNACKS:							
DRINKS:							
TOTAL							

WATER (8-oz glasses OR 2 litres of water a day):	Yes ⨯	No ⨯

TOTAL SLEEP / REST HOURS	NIGHT	DAY	TOTAL

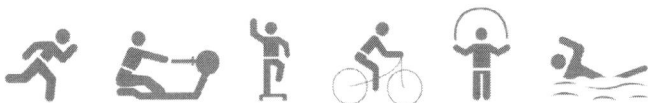

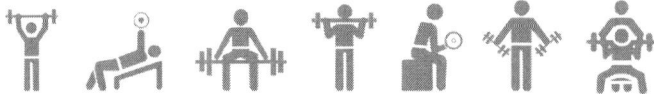

Day/Date: *Time/Duration:*

WEIGHT TRAINING

Muscle Group(s)	Chest		Shoulders		Back		Arms		Rest between Sets	Legs	Abs
EXERCISE	Set 1		Set 2		Set 3		Set 4			Set 5 or the Set with Max. Wt./Reps	
	Weight	Reps	Weight	Reps	Weight	Reps	Weight	Reps		Weight	Reps

CARDIO & STRETCHING   Time/Duration: NOTES

EXERCISE / LEVEL	Time/ Duration		Distance		Calories		Ideas/goals for next session:
	Goal	Actual	Goal	Actual	Goal	Actual	

DIET & SLEEP

MEALS	Protein	Carbs	Total Fat	Sugars	Sodium/Salt	Fiber	Calories
BREAKFAST:							
LUNCH:							
DINNER:							
SNACKS:							
DRINKS:							
TOTAL							

WATER (8-oz glasses OR 2 litres of water a day):   Yes ✗   No ✗

TOTAL SLEEP / REST HOURS	NIGHT	DAY	TOTAL

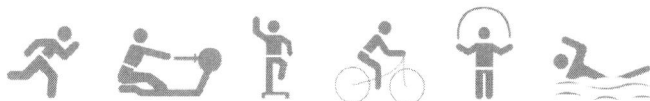

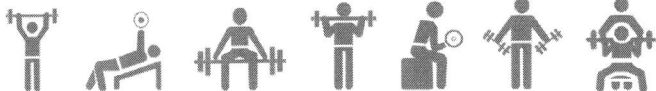

Day/Date: Time/Duration:

WEIGHT TRAINING

Muscle Group(s)	Chest		Shoulders		Back		Arms		Rest between Sets	Legs Abs Set 5 or the Set with Max. Wt./Reps	
	Set 1		Set 2		Set 3		Set 4				
EXERCISE	Weight	Reps	Weight	Reps	Weight	Reps	Weight	Reps		Weight	Reps

CARDIO & STRETCHING   Time/Duration: NOTES

EXERCISE / LEVEL	Time/ Duration		Distance		Calories		Ideas/goals for next session:
	Goal	Actual	Goal	Actual	Goal	Actual	

DIET & SLEEP

MEALS	Protein	Carbs	Total Fat	Sugars	Sodium/ Salt	Fiber	Calories
BREAKFAST:							
LUNCH:							
DINNER:							
SNACKS:							
DRINKS:							
TOTAL							

WATER (8-oz glasses OR 2 litres of water a day):		Yes	☓	No	☓
TOTAL SLEEP / REST HOURS	NIGHT		DAY		TOTAL

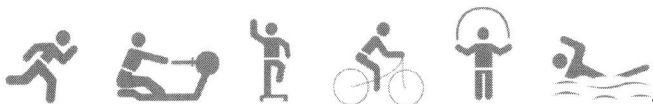

WEIGHT TRAINING

Day/Date: Time/Duration:

Muscle Group(s)   Chest   Shoulders   Back   Arms   Legs   Abs

EXERCISE	Set 1 Weight	Reps	Set 2 Weight	Reps	Set 3 Weight	Reps	Set 4 Weight	Reps	Rest between Sets	Set 5 or the Set with Max. Wt./Reps Weight	Reps

CARDIO & STRETCHING   Time/Duration: NOTES

Ideas/goals for next session:

EXERCISE / LEVEL	Time/Duration Goal	Actual	Distance Goal	Actual	Calories Goal	Actual

DIET & SLEEP

MEALS	Protein	Carbs	Total Fat	Sugars	Sodium/ Salt	Fiber	Calories
BREAKFAST:							
LUNCH:							
DINNER:							
SNACKS:							
DRINKS:							
TOTAL							

WATER (8-oz glasses OR 2 litres of water a day):	Yes ✕	No ✕

TOTAL SLEEP / REST HOURS	NIGHT	DAY	TOTAL

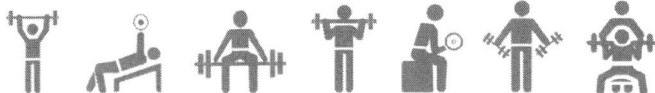

WEIGHT TRAINING

Day/Date: Time/Duration:

Muscle Group(s)	Chest		Shoulders		Back		Arms		Rest between Sets	Legs Abs Set 5 or the Set with Max. Wt./Reps	
	Set 1		Set 2		Set 3		Set 4				
EXERCISE	Weight	Reps	Weight	Reps	Weight	Reps	Weight	Reps		Weight	Reps

CARDIO & STRETCHING   Time/Duration: NOTES

Ideas/goals for next session:

EXERCISE / LEVEL	Time/ Duration		Distance		Calories	
	Goal	Actual	Goal	Actual	Goal	Actual

DIET & SLEEP

MEALS	Protein	Carbs	Total Fat	Sugars	Sodium/ Salt	Fiber	Calories
BREAKFAST:							
LUNCH:							
DINNER:							
SNACKS:							
DRINKS:							
TOTAL							

WATER (8-oz glasses OR 2 litres of water a day):		Yes ✕	No ✕
TOTAL SLEEP / REST HOURS	NIGHT	DAY	TOTAL

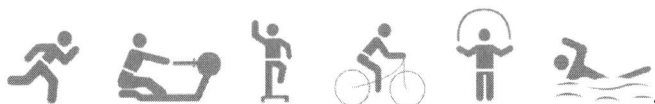

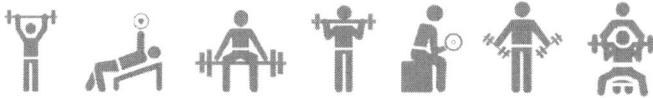

Day/Date: _____   Time/Duration: _____

WEIGHT TRAINING

Muscle Group(s)   **Chest**   **Shoulders**   **Back**   **Arms**   **Legs   Abs**

EXERCISE	Set 1		Set 2		Set 3		Set 4		Rest between Sets	Set 5 or the Set with Max. Wt./Reps	
	Weight	Reps	Weight	Reps	Weight	Reps	Weight	Reps		Weight	Reps

CARDIO & STRETCHING   Time/Duration: _____   NOTES

EXERCISE / LEVEL	Time/ Duration		Distance		Calories		Ideas/goals for next session:
	Goal	Actual	Goal	Actual	Goal	Actual	

DIET & SLEEP

MEALS	Protein	Carbs	Total Fat	Sugars	Sodium/ Salt	Fiber	Calories
BREAKFAST:							
LUNCH:							
DINNER:							
SNACKS:							
DRINKS:							
TOTAL							

WATER (8-oz glasses OR 2 litres of water a day):		Yes ✕	No ✕

TOTAL SLEEP / REST HOURS	NIGHT	DAY	TOTAL

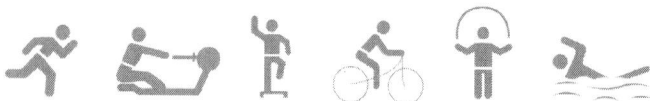

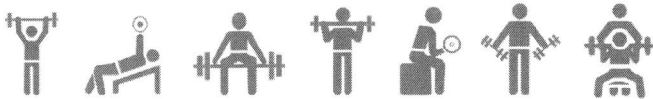

WEIGHT TRAINING

Day/Date: Time/Duration:

Muscle Group(s)	Chest		Shoulders		Back		Arms		Rest between Sets	Legs Abs Set 5 or the Set with Max. Wt./Reps	
EXERCISE	Set 1		Set 2		Set 3		Set 4				
	Weight	Reps	Weight	Reps	Weight	Reps	Weight	Reps		Weight	Reps

CARDIO & STRETCHING   Time/Duration: *NOTES*

Ideas/goals for next session:

EXERCISE / LEVEL	Time/Duration		Distance		Calories	
	Goal	Actual	Goal	Actual	Goal	Actual

DIET & SLEEP

MEALS	Protein	Carbs	Total Fat	Sugars	Sodium/ Salt	Fiber	Calories
BREAKFAST:							
LUNCH:							
DINNER:							
SNACKS:							
DRINKS:							
TOTAL							

WATER (8-oz glasses OR 2 litres of water a day):		Yes	✗	No	✗

	NIGHT	DAY	TOTAL
TOTAL SLEEP / REST HOURS			

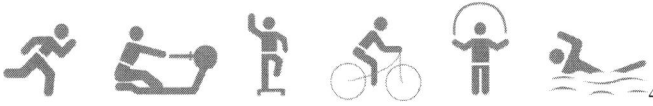

WEIGHT TRAINING

Day/Date: Time/Duration:

Muscle Group(s)   Chest   Shoulders   Back   Arms   Legs   Abs

EXERCISE	Set 1 Weight	Set 1 Reps	Set 2 Weight	Set 2 Reps	Set 3 Weight	Set 3 Reps	Set 4 Weight	Set 4 Reps	Rest between Sets	Set 5 or the Set with Max. Wt./Reps Weight	Reps

CARDIO & STRETCHING   Time/Duration: NOTES

EXERCISE / LEVEL	Time/ Duration Goal	Actual	Distance Goal	Actual	Calories Goal	Actual	Ideas/goals for next session:

DIET & SLEEP

MEALS	Protein	Carbs	Total Fat	Sugars	Sodium/ Salt	Fiber	Calories
BREAKFAST:							
LUNCH:							
DINNER:							
SNACKS:							
DRINKS:							
TOTAL							

WATER (8-oz glasses OR 2 litres of water a day):   Yes   No

TOTAL SLEEP / REST HOURS	NIGHT	DAY	TOTAL

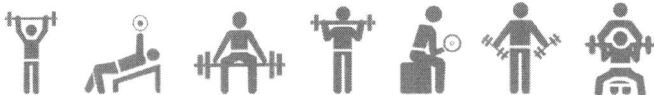

Day/Date: *Time/Duration:*

WEIGHT TRAINING

Muscle Group(s)   **Chest**   **Shoulders**   **Back**   **Arms**   **Legs**   **Abs**

EXERCISE	Set 1 Weight	Set 1 Reps	Set 2 Weight	Set 2 Reps	Set 3 Weight	Set 3 Reps	Set 4 Weight	Set 4 Reps	Rest between Sets	Set 5 or the Set with Max. Wt./Reps Weight	Reps

CARDIO & STRETCHING	*Time/Duration:*						*NOTES*

Ideas/goals for next session:

EXERCISE / LEVEL	Time/ Duration Goal	Actual	Distance Goal	Actual	Calories Goal	Actual

DIET & SLEEP

MEALS	Protein	Carbs	Total Fat	Sugars	Sodium/ Salt	Fiber	Calories
BREAKFAST:							
LUNCH:							
DINNER:							
SNACKS:							
DRINKS:							
TOTAL							

WATER (8-oz glasses OR 2 litres of water a day):		Yes	✕	No	✕

TOTAL SLEEP / REST HOURS	NIGHT	DAY	TOTAL

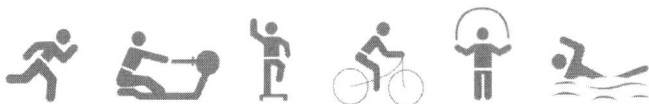

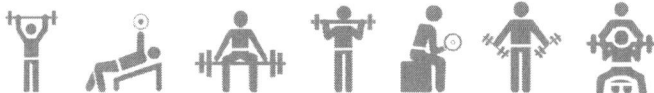

Day/Date: _____   **Time/Duration:** _____

WEIGHT TRAINING

Muscle Group(s)   **Chest   Shoulders   Back   Arms   Legs   Abs**

EXERCISE	Set 1 Weight	Set 1 Reps	Set 2 Weight	Set 2 Reps	Set 3 Weight	Set 3 Reps	Set 4 Weight	Set 4 Reps	Rest between Sets	Set 5 or the Set with Max. Wt./Reps Weight	Reps

CARDIO & STRETCHING   Time/Duration: _____   NOTES

Ideas/goals for next session:

EXERCISE / LEVEL	Time/Duration Goal	Time/Duration Actual	Distance Goal	Distance Actual	Calories Goal	Calories Actual

DIET & SLEEP

MEALS	Protein	Carbs	Total Fat	Sugars	Sodium/ Salt	Fiber	Calories
BREAKFAST:							
LUNCH:							
DINNER:							
SNACKS:							
DRINKS:							
TOTAL							

WATER (8-oz glasses OR 2 litres of water a day):	Yes ✕	No ✕

TOTAL SLEEP / REST HOURS	NIGHT	DAY	TOTAL

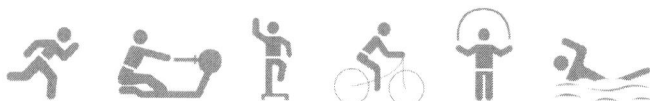

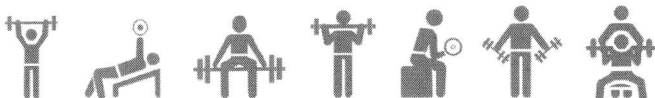

Day/Date: **Time/Duration:**

WEIGHT TRAINING

Muscle Group(s)   **Chest**   **Shoulders**   **Back**   **Arms**   **Legs**   **Abs**

EXERCISE	Set 1 Weight	Set 1 Reps	Set 2 Weight	Set 2 Reps	Set 3 Weight	Set 3 Reps	Set 4 Weight	Set 4 Reps	Rest between Sets	Set 5 or the Set with Max. Wt./Reps Weight	Reps

CARDIO & STRETCHING   **Time/Duration:**   *NOTES*

EXERCISE / LEVEL	Time/Duration Goal	Time/Duration Actual	Distance Goal	Distance Actual	Calories Goal	Calories Actual	Ideas/goals for next session:

DIET & SLEEP

MEALS	Protein	Carbs	Total Fat	Sugars	Sodium/Salt	Fiber	Calories
BREAKFAST:							
LUNCH:							
DINNER:							
SNACKS:							
DRINKS:							
TOTAL							

WATER (8-oz glasses OR 2 litres of water a day):		Yes	✕	No	✕

TOTAL SLEEP / REST HOURS	NIGHT	DAY	TOTAL

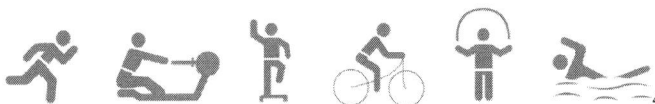

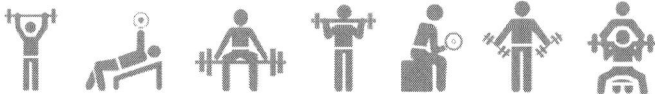

	Day/Date:		Time/Duration:

WEIGHT TRAINING

Muscle Group(s)	Chest		Shoulders		Back		Arms			Legs	Abs
	Set 1		Set 2		Set 3		Set 4		Rest between Sets	Set 5 or the Set with Max. Wt./Reps	
EXERCISE	Weight	Reps	Weight	Reps	Weight	Reps	Weight	Reps		Weight	Reps

CARDIO & STRETCHING   Time/Duration: NOTES

	Time/Duration		Distance		Calories		Ideas/goals for next session:
EXERCISE / LEVEL	Goal	Actual	Goal	Actual	Goal	Actual	

DIET & SLEEP

MEALS	Protein	Carbs	Total Fat	Sugars	Sodium/Salt	Fiber	Calories
BREAKFAST:							
LUNCH:							
DINNER:							
SNACKS:							
DRINKS:							
TOTAL							

WATER (8-oz glasses OR 2 litres of water a day):	Yes	No

TOTAL SLEEP / REST HOURS	NIGHT	DAY	TOTAL

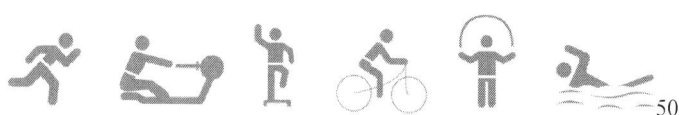

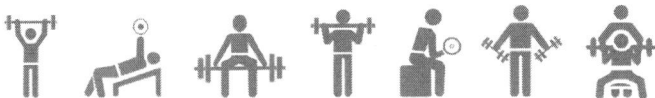

Day/Date: _____   **Time/Duration:** _____

WEIGHT TRAINING

Muscle Group(s) Chest   Shoulders   Back   Arms   Legs   Abs

EXERCISE	Set 1 Weight	Set 1 Reps	Set 2 Weight	Set 2 Reps	Set 3 Weight	Set 3 Reps	Set 4 Weight	Set 4 Reps	Rest between Sets	Set 5 or the Set with Max. Wt./Reps Weight	Reps

CARDIO & STRETCHING   Time/Duration: _____   *NOTES*

Ideas/goals for next session:

EXERCISE / LEVEL	Time/Duration Goal	Actual	Distance Goal	Actual	Calories Goal	Actual

DIET & SLEEP

MEALS	Protein	Carbs	Total Fat	Sugars	Sodium/Salt	Fiber	Calories
BREAKFAST:							
LUNCH:							
DINNER:							
SNACKS:							
DRINKS:							
TOTAL							

WATER (8-oz glasses OR 2 litres of water a day):   Yes ✕   No ✕

TOTAL SLEEP / REST HOURS	NIGHT	DAY	TOTAL

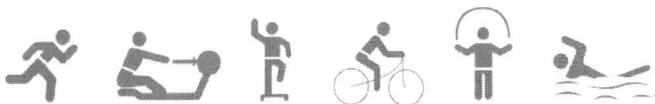

Day/Date: _____ Time/Duration: _____

WEIGHT TRAINING

Muscle Group(s) Chest   Shoulders   Back   Arms   Legs   Abs

EXERCISE	Set 1 Weight	Set 1 Reps	Set 2 Weight	Set 2 Reps	Set 3 Weight	Set 3 Reps	Set 4 Weight	Set 4 Reps	Rest between Sets	Set 5 or the Set with Max. Wt./Reps Weight	Reps

CARDIO & STRETCHING   Time/Duration: _____   NOTES

Ideas/goals for next session:

EXERCISE / LEVEL	Time/ Duration Goal	Actual	Distance Goal	Actual	Calories Goal	Actual

DIET & SLEEP

MEALS	Protein	Carbs	Total Fat	Sugars	Sodium/ Salt	Fiber	Calories
BREAKFAST:							
LUNCH:							
DINNER:							
SNACKS:							
DRINKS:							
TOTAL							

WATER (8-oz glasses OR 2 litres of water a day):   Yes ✕   No ✕

TOTAL SLEEP / REST HOURS	NIGHT	DAY	TOTAL

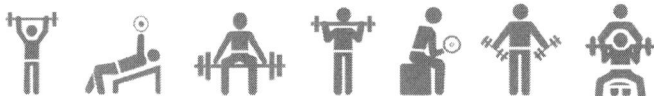

WEIGHT TRAINING

Day/Date: Time/Duration:

Muscle Group(s)   Chest   Shoulders   Back   Arms   Legs   Abs

EXERCISE	Set 1		Set 2		Set 3		Set 4		Rest between Sets	Set 5 or the Set with Max. Wt./Reps	
	Weight	Reps	Weight	Reps	Weight	Reps	Weight	Reps		Weight	Reps

CARDIO & STRETCHING   Time/Duration: NOTES

EXERCISE / LEVEL	Time/ Duration		Distance		Calories		Ideas/goals for next session:
	Goal	Actual	Goal	Actual	Goal	Actual	

DIET & SLEEP

MEALS	Protein	Carbs	Total Fat	Sugars	Sodium/Salt	Fiber	Calories
BREAKFAST:							
LUNCH:							
DINNER:							
SNACKS:							
DRINKS:							
TOTAL							

WATER (8-oz glasses OR 2 litres of water a day):		Yes ✗ No ✗

TOTAL SLEEP / REST HOURS	NIGHT	DAY	TOTAL

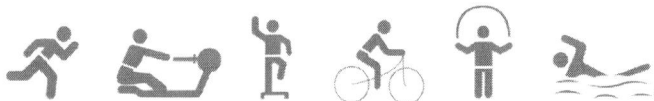

53

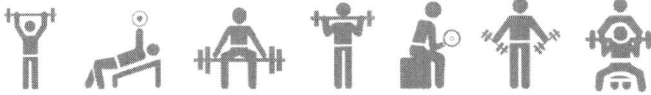

Day/Date: Time/Duration:

WEIGHT TRAINING

Muscle Group(s)   Chest   Shoulders   Back   Arms   Legs   Abs

EXERCISE	Set 1		Set 2		Set 3		Set 4		Rest between Sets	Set 5 or the Set with Max. Wt./Reps	
	Weight	Reps	Weight	Reps	Weight	Reps	Weight	Reps		Weight	Reps

CARDIO & STRETCHING   Time/Duration: NOTES

EXERCISE / LEVEL	Time/ Duration		Distance		Calories		Ideas/goals for next session:
	Goal	Actual	Goal	Actual	Goal	Actual	

DIET & SLEEP

MEALS	Protein	Carbs	Total Fat	Sugars	Sodium/ Salt	Fiber	Calories
BREAKFAST:							
LUNCH:							
DINNER:							
SNACKS:							
DRINKS:							
TOTAL							

WATER (8-oz glasses OR 2 litres of water a day):		Yes	✕	No	✕

TOTAL SLEEP / REST HOURS	NIGHT	DAY	TOTAL

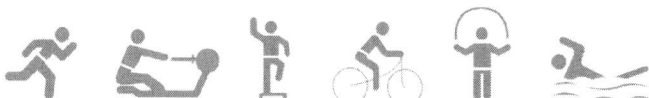

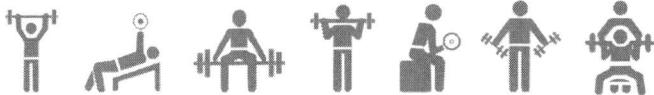

WEIGHT TRAINING

Day/Date: _____   Time/Duration: _____

Muscle Group(s)	Chest		Shoulders		Back		Arms			Legs	Abs

| | Set 1 | | Set 2 | | Set 3 | | Set 4 | | Rest between Sets | Set 5 or the Set with Max. Wt./Reps | |
EXERCISE	Weight	Reps	Weight	Reps	Weight	Reps	Weight	Reps		Weight	Reps

CARDIO & STRETCHING   Time/Duration: _____   NOTES

Ideas/goals for next session:

EXERCISE / LEVEL	Time/Duration		Distance		Calories	
	Goal	Actual	Goal	Actual	Goal	Actual

DIET & SLEEP

MEALS	Protein	Carbs	Total Fat	Sugars	Sodium/Salt	Fiber	Calories
BREAKFAST:							
LUNCH:							
DINNER:							
SNACKS:							
DRINKS:							
TOTAL							

WATER (8-oz glasses OR 2 litres of water a day):   Yes ☒   No ☒

TOTAL SLEEP / REST HOURS	NIGHT	DAY	TOTAL

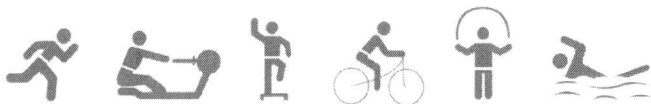

	Day/Date:		Time/Duration:

WEIGHT TRAINING

Muscle Group(s)	Chest		Shoulders		Back		Arms		Rest between Sets	Legs Abs Set 5 or the Set with Max. Wt./Reps	
	Set 1		Set 2		Set 3		Set 4				
EXERCISE	Weight	Reps	Weight	Reps	Weight	Reps	Weight	Reps		Weight	Reps

CARDIO & STRETCHING   Time/Duration:

EXERCISE / LEVEL	Time/Duration		Distance		Calories		NOTES Ideas/goals for next session:
	Goal	Actual	Goal	Actual	Goal	Actual	

DIET & SLEEP

MEALS	Protein	Carbs	Total Fat	Sugars	Sodium/Salt	Fiber	Calories
BREAKFAST:							
LUNCH:							
DINNER:							
SNACKS:							
DRINKS:							
TOTAL							

WATER (8-oz glasses OR 2 litres of water a day):   Yes   ×   No   ×

TOTAL SLEEP / REST HOURS	NIGHT	DAY	TOTAL

56

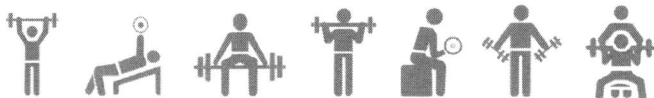

Day/Date: _____   Time/Duration: _____

WEIGHT TRAINING

Muscle Group(s) *Chest*   *Shoulders*   *Back*   *Arms*   *Legs*   *Abs*

EXERCISE	Set 1		Set 2		Set 3		Set 4		Rest between Sets	Set 5 or the Set with Max. Wt./Reps	
	Weight	Reps	Weight	Reps	Weight	Reps	Weight	Reps		Weight	Reps

CARDIO & STRETCHING   Time/Duration: _____   NOTES

Ideas/goals for next session:

EXERCISE / LEVEL	Time/ Duration		Distance		Calories	
	Goal	Actual	Goal	Actual	Goal	Actual

DIET & SLEEP

MEALS	Protein	Carbs	Total Fat	Sugars	Sodium/ Salt	Fiber	Calories
BREAKFAST:							
LUNCH:							
DINNER:							
SNACKS:							
DRINKS:							
TOTAL							

WATER (8-oz glasses OR 2 litres of water a day):		Yes ✕	No ✕

TOTAL SLEEP / REST HOURS	NIGHT	DAY	TOTAL

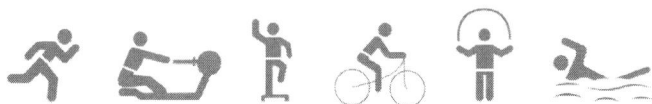

Day/Date: _____   Time/Duration: _____

WEIGHT TRAINING

Muscle Group(s)	Chest		Shoulders		Back		Arms		Rest between Sets	Legs Abs	
	Set 1		Set 2		Set 3		Set 4			Set 5 or the Set with Max. Wt./Reps	
EXERCISE	Weight	Reps	Weight	Reps	Weight	Reps	Weight	Reps		Weight	Reps

CARDIO & STRETCHING   Time/Duration: _____   NOTES

EXERCISE / LEVEL	Time/ Duration		Distance		Calories		Ideas/goals for next session:
	Goal	Actual	Goal	Actual	Goal	Actual	

DIET & SLEEP

MEALS	Protein	Carbs	Total Fat	Sugars	Sodium/ Salt	Fiber	Calories
BREAKFAST:							
LUNCH:							
DINNER:							
SNACKS:							
DRINKS:							
TOTAL							

WATER (8-oz glasses OR 2 litres of water a day):   Yes ☒   No ☒

TOTAL SLEEP / REST HOURS	NIGHT	DAY	TOTAL

58

WEIGHT TRAINING

Day/Date: *Time/Duration:*

Muscle Group(s)   Chest   Shoulders   Back   Arms   Legs   Abs

EXERCISE	Set 1 Weight	Set 1 Reps	Set 2 Weight	Set 2 Reps	Set 3 Weight	Set 3 Reps	Set 4 Weight	Set 4 Reps	Rest between Sets	Set 5 or the Set with Max. Wt./Reps Weight	Reps

CARDIO & STRETCHING   Time/Duration: NOTES

Ideas/goals for next session:

EXERCISE / LEVEL	Time/Duration Goal	Actual	Distance Goal	Actual	Calories Goal	Actual

DIET & SLEEP

MEALS	Protein	Carbs	Total Fat	Sugars	Sodium/Salt	Fiber	Calories
BREAKFAST:							
LUNCH:							
DINNER:							
SNACKS:							
DRINKS:							
TOTAL							

WATER (8-oz glasses OR 2 litres of water a day):   Yes   ✕   No   ✕

TOTAL SLEEP / REST HOURS	NIGHT	DAY	TOTAL

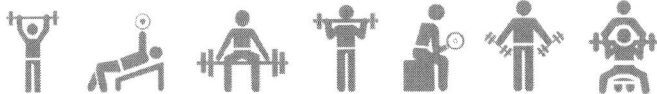

WEIGHT TRAINING

Day/Date: Time/Duration:

Muscle Group(s)	Chest		Shoulders		Back		Arms		Rest between Sets	Legs Abs Set 5 or the Set with Max. Wt./Reps	
	Set 1		Set 2		Set 3		Set 4				
EXERCISE	Weight	Reps	Weight	Reps	Weight	Reps	Weight	Reps		Weight	Reps

CARDIO & STRETCHING Time/Duration: NOTES

EXERCISE / LEVEL	Time/ Duration		Distance		Calories		Ideas/goals for next session:
	Goal	Actual	Goal	Actual	Goal	Actual	

DIET & SLEEP

MEALS	Protein	Carbs	Total Fat	Sugars	Sodium/ Salt	Fiber	Calories
BREAKFAST:							
LUNCH:							
DINNER:							
SNACKS:							
DRINKS:							
TOTAL							

WATER (8-oz glasses OR 2 litres of water a day):		Yes		No	

TOTAL SLEEP / REST HOURS	NIGHT	DAY	TOTAL

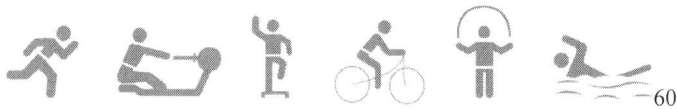

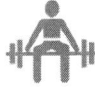

Day/Date: _____   Time/Duration: _____

WEIGHT TRAINING

Muscle Group(s)	Chest		Shoulders		Back		Arms		Legs	Abs
	Set 1		Set 2		Set 3		Set 4		Rest between Sets	Set 5 or the Set with Max. Wt./Reps
EXERCISE	Weight	Reps	Weight	Reps	Weight	Reps	Weight	Reps		Weight	Reps

CARDIO & STRETCHING   Time/Duration: _____

	Time/ Duration		Distance		Calories		NOTES — Ideas/goals for next session:
EXERCISE / LEVEL	Goal	Actual	Goal	Actual	Goal	Actual	

DIET & SLEEP

MEALS	Protein	Carbs	Total Fat	Sugars	Sodium/ Salt	Fiber	Calories
BREAKFAST:							
LUNCH:							
DINNER:							
SNACKS:							
DRINKS:							
TOTAL							

WATER (8-oz glasses OR 2 litres of water a day):		Yes ✕	No ✕

TOTAL SLEEP / REST HOURS	NIGHT	DAY	TOTAL

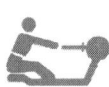 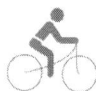 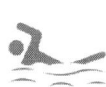

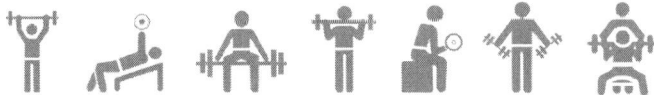

WEIGHT TRAINING

Day/Date: Time/Duration:

Muscle Group(s)	Chest		Shoulders		Back		Arms		Rest between Sets	Set 5 or the Set with Max. Wt./Reps	
	Set 1		Set 2		Set 3		Set 4				
EXERCISE	Weight	Reps	Weight	Reps	Weight	Reps	Weight	Reps		Weight	Reps

CARDIO & STRETCHING   Time/Duration: NOTES

EXERCISE / LEVEL	Time/Duration		Distance		Calories		Ideas/goals for next session:
	Goal	Actual	Goal	Actual	Goal	Actual	

DIET & SLEEP

MEALS	Protein	Carbs	Total Fat	Sugars	Sodium/Salt	Fiber	Calories
BREAKFAST:							
LUNCH:							
DINNER:							
SNACKS:							
DRINKS:							
TOTAL							

WATER (8-oz glasses OR 2 litres of water a day):   Yes   ✕   No   ✕

TOTAL SLEEP / REST HOURS	NIGHT	DAY	TOTAL

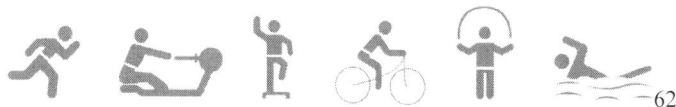

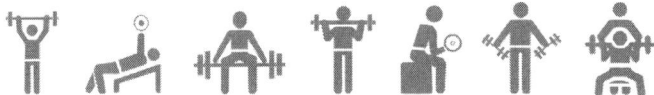

Day/Date: _____   **Time/Duration:** _____

WEIGHT TRAINING

Muscle Group(s)   Chest   Shoulders   Back   Arms   Legs   Abs

EXERCISE	Set 1 Weight	Set 1 Reps	Set 2 Weight	Set 2 Reps	Set 3 Weight	Set 3 Reps	Set 4 Weight	Set 4 Reps	Rest between Sets	Set 5 or the Set with Max. Wt./Reps Weight	Reps

CARDIO & STRETCHING   Time/Duration: _____   *NOTES*

Ideas/goals for next session:

EXERCISE / LEVEL	Time/Duration Goal	Actual	Distance Goal	Actual	Calories Goal	Actual

DIET & SLEEP

MEALS	Protein	Carbs	Total Fat	Sugars	Sodium/Salt	Fiber	Calories
BREAKFAST:							
LUNCH:							
DINNER:							
SNACKS:							
DRINKS:							
TOTAL							

WATER (8-oz glasses OR 2 litres of water a day):   Yes ☒   No ☒

TOTAL SLEEP / REST HOURS	NIGHT	DAY	TOTAL

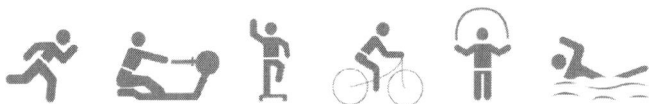

Day/Date: _____   Time/Duration: _____

WEIGHT TRAINING

Muscle Group(s)	Chest		Shoulders		Back		Arms		Rest between Sets	Legs Abs	
	Set 1		Set 2		Set 3		Set 4			Set 5 or the Set with Max. Wt./Reps	
EXERCISE	Weight	Reps	Weight	Reps	Weight	Reps	Weight	Reps		Weight	Reps

CARDIO & STRETCHING   Time/Duration: _____   NOTES

EXERCISE / LEVEL	Time/ Duration		Distance		Calories		Ideas/goals for next session:
	Goal	Actual	Goal	Actual	Goal	Actual	

DIET & SLEEP

MEALS	Protein	Carbs	Total Fat	Sugars	Sodium/ Salt	Fiber	Calories
BREAKFAST:							
LUNCH:							
DINNER:							
SNACKS:							
DRINKS:							
TOTAL							

WATER (8-oz glasses OR 2 litres of water a day):		Yes ✕		No ✕

TOTAL SLEEP / REST HOURS	NIGHT	DAY	TOTAL

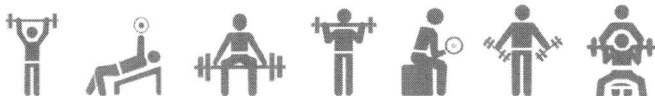

WEIGHT TRAINING

Day/Date: Time/Duration:

Muscle Group(s)	Chest		Shoulders		Back		Arms		Rest between Sets	Legs Abs Set 5 or the Set with Max. Wt./Reps	
	Set 1		Set 2		Set 3		Set 4				
EXERCISE	Weight	Reps	Weight	Reps	Weight	Reps	Weight	Reps		Weight	Reps

CARDIO & STRETCHING   Time/Duration: NOTES

EXERCISE / LEVEL	Time/ Duration		Distance		Calories		Ideas/goals for next session:
	Goal	Actual	Goal	Actual	Goal	Actual	

DIET & SLEEP

MEALS	Protein	Carbs	Total Fat	Sugars	Sodium/ Salt	Fiber	Calories
BREAKFAST:							
LUNCH:							
DINNER:							
SNACKS:							
DRINKS:							
TOTAL							

WATER (8-oz glasses OR 2 litres of water a day):		Yes ✕ No ✕	
TOTAL SLEEP / REST HOURS	**NIGHT**	**DAY**	**TOTAL**

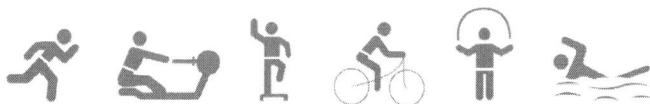

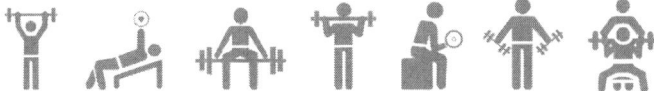

Day/Date: _____ **Time/Duration:** _____

WEIGHT TRAINING

Muscle Group(s) **Chest** **Shoulders** **Back** **Arms** **Legs** **Abs**

EXERCISE	Set 1		Set 2		Set 3		Set 4		Rest between Sets	Set 5 or the Set with Max. Wt./Reps	
	Weight	Reps	Weight	Reps	Weight	Reps	Weight	Reps		Weight	Reps

CARDIO & STRETCHING   Time/Duration: _____   NOTES

EXERCISE / LEVEL	Time/Duration		Distance		Calories		Ideas/goals for next session:
	Goal	Actual	Goal	Actual	Goal	Actual	

DIET & SLEEP

MEALS	Protein	Carbs	Total Fat	Sugars	Sodium/Salt	Fiber	Calories
BREAKFAST:							
LUNCH:							
DINNER:							
SNACKS:							
DRINKS:							
TOTAL							

WATER (8-oz glasses OR 2 litres of water a day):   Yes ✕   No ✕

TOTAL SLEEP / REST HOURS	NIGHT	DAY	TOTAL

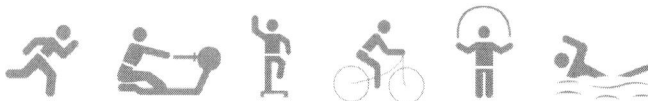

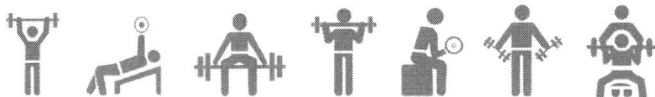

WEIGHT TRAINING

Day/Date: Time/Duration:

Muscle Group(s)	Chest		Shoulders		Back		Arms		Rest between Sets	Legs Abs Set 5 or the Set with Max. Wt./Reps	
	Set 1		Set 2		Set 3		Set 4				
EXERCISE	Weight	Reps	Weight	Reps	Weight	Reps	Weight	Reps		Weight	Reps

CARDIO & STRETCHING   Time/Duration: NOTES

Ideas/goals for next session:

EXERCISE / LEVEL	Time/ Duration		Distance		Calories	
	Goal	Actual	Goal	Actual	Goal	Actual

DIET & SLEEP

MEALS	Protein	Carbs	Total Fat	Sugars	Sodium/Salt	Fiber	Calories
BREAKFAST:							
LUNCH:							
DINNER:							
SNACKS:							
DRINKS:							
TOTAL							

WATER (8-oz glasses OR 2 litres of water a day):		Yes ×	No ×

TOTAL SLEEP / REST HOURS	NIGHT	DAY	TOTAL

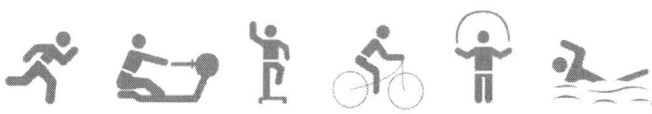

WEIGHT TRAINING

Day/Date: _____   Time/Duration: _____

Muscle Group(s)	Chest		Shoulders		Back		Arms		Rest between Sets	Legs	Abs
										Set 5 or the Set with Max. Wt./Reps	
	Set 1		Set 2		Set 3		Set 4				
EXERCISE	Weight	Reps	Weight	Reps	Weight	Reps	Weight	Reps		Weight	Reps

CARDIO & STRETCHING   Time/Duration: _____   NOTES

| EXERCISE / LEVEL | Time/ Duration | | Distance | | Calories | |
	Goal	Actual	Goal	Actual	Goal	Actual

Ideas/goals for next session:

DIET & SLEEP

MEALS	Protein	Carbs	Total Fat	Sugars	Sodium/ Salt	Fiber	Calories
BREAKFAST:							
LUNCH:							
DINNER:							
SNACKS:							
DRINKS:							
TOTAL							

WATER (8-oz glasses OR 2 litres of water a day):   Yes ✕   No ✕

TOTAL SLEEP / REST HOURS	NIGHT	DAY	TOTAL

68

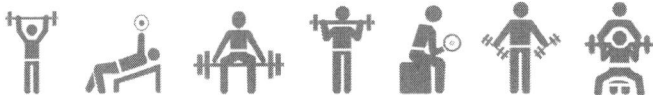

WEIGHT TRAINING

Day/Date: _____   Time/Duration: _____

Muscle Group(s)	Chest		Shoulders		Back		Arms		Rest between Sets	Legs	Abs
	Set 1		Set 2		Set 3		Set 4			Set 5 or the Set with Max. Wt./Reps	
EXERCISE	Weight	Reps	Weight	Reps	Weight	Reps	Weight	Reps		Weight	Reps

CARDIO & STRETCHING   Time/Duration: _____   NOTES

Ideas/goals for next session:

EXERCISE / LEVEL	Time/ Duration		Distance		Calories	
	Goal	Actual	Goal	Actual	Goal	Actual

DIET & SLEEP

MEALS	Protein	Carbs	Total Fat	Sugars	Sodium/Salt	Fiber	Calories
BREAKFAST:							
LUNCH:							
DINNER:							
SNACKS:							
DRINKS:							
TOTAL							

WATER (8-oz glasses OR 2 litres of water a day):   Yes ✕   No ✕

TOTAL SLEEP / REST HOURS	NIGHT	DAY	TOTAL

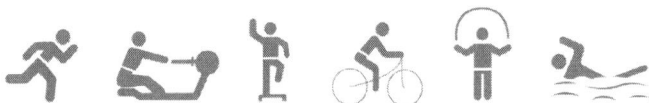

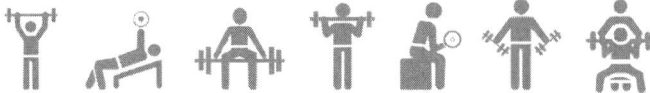

WEIGHT TRAINING

Day/Date: _____   Time/Duration: _____

Muscle Group(s)	Chest		Shoulders		Back		Arms		Rest between Sets	Legs Abs — Set 5 or the Set with Max. Wt./Reps	
	Set 1		Set 2		Set 3		Set 4				
EXERCISE	Weight	Reps	Weight	Reps	Weight	Reps	Weight	Reps		Weight	Reps

CARDIO & STRETCHING   Time/Duration: _____   NOTES

EXERCISE / LEVEL	Time/ Duration		Distance		Calories		Ideas/goals for next session:
	Goal	Actual	Goal	Actual	Goal	Actual	

DIET & SLEEP

MEALS	Protein	Carbs	Total Fat	Sugars	Sodium/Salt	Fiber	Calories
BREAKFAST:							
LUNCH:							
DINNER:							
SNACKS:							
DRINKS:							
TOTAL							

WATER (8-oz glasses OR 2 litres of water a day):   Yes   ✕   No   ✕

TOTAL SLEEP / REST HOURS	NIGHT	DAY	TOTAL

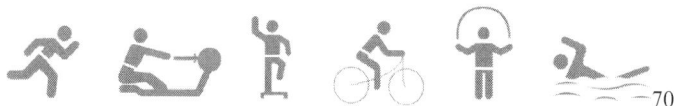

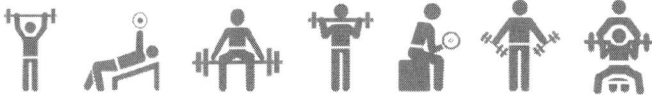

WEIGHT TRAINING

Day/Date: Time/Duration:

Muscle Group(s)	Chest		Shoulders		Back		Arms		Rest between Sets	Legs	Abs
	Set 1		Set 2		Set 3		Set 4			Set 5 or the Set with Max. Wt./Reps	
EXERCISE	Weight	Reps	Weight	Reps	Weight	Reps	Weight	Reps		Weight	Reps

CARDIO & STRETCHING

Time/Duration: **NOTES**

EXERCISE / LEVEL	Time/Duration		Distance		Calories		Ideas/goals for next session:
	Goal	Actual	Goal	Actual	Goal	Actual	

DIET & SLEEP

MEALS	Protein	Carbs	Total Fat	Sugars	Sodium/ Salt	Fiber	Calories
BREAKFAST:							
LUNCH:							
DINNER:							
SNACKS:							
DRINKS:							
TOTAL							

WATER (8-oz glasses OR 2 litres of water a day):		Yes ✕ No ✕	
TOTAL SLEEP / REST HOURS	**NIGHT**	**DAY**	**TOTAL**

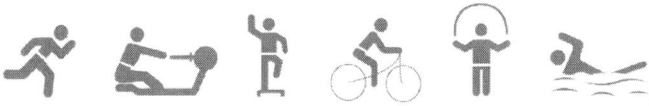

71

Day/Date: _____   Time/Duration: _____

WEIGHT TRAINING

Muscle Group(s) Chest   Shoulders   Back   Arms   Legs   Abs

EXERCISE	Set 1 Weight	Set 1 Reps	Set 2 Weight	Set 2 Reps	Set 3 Weight	Set 3 Reps	Set 4 Weight	Set 4 Reps	Rest between Sets	Set 5 or the Set with Max. Wt./Reps Weight	Reps

CARDIO & STRETCHING   Time/Duration: _____   NOTES

Ideas/goals for next session:

EXERCISE / LEVEL	Time/ Duration Goal	Actual	Distance Goal	Actual	Calories Goal	Actual

DIET & SLEEP

MEALS	Protein	Carbs	Total Fat	Sugars	Sodium/ Salt	Fiber	Calories
BREAKFAST:							
LUNCH:							
DINNER:							
SNACKS:							
DRINKS:							
TOTAL							

WATER (8-oz glasses OR 2 litres of water a day):   Yes ✕   No ✕

TOTAL SLEEP / REST HOURS	NIGHT	DAY	TOTAL

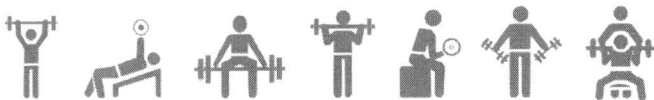

Day/Date: _____   Time/Duration: _____

WEIGHT TRAINING

Muscle Group(s)   **Chest   Shoulders   Back   Arms   Legs   Abs**

EXERCISE	Set 1 Weight	Set 1 Reps	Set 2 Weight	Set 2 Reps	Set 3 Weight	Set 3 Reps	Set 4 Weight	Set 4 Reps	Rest between Sets	Set 5 or the Set with Max. Wt./Reps Weight	Reps

CARDIO & STRETCHING   Time/Duration: _____   NOTES

EXERCISE / LEVEL	Time/Duration Goal	Actual	Distance Goal	Actual	Calories Goal	Actual	Ideas/goals for next session:

DIET & SLEEP

MEALS	Protein	Carbs	Total Fat	Sugars	Sodium/Salt	Fiber	Calories
BREAKFAST:							
LUNCH:							
DINNER:							
SNACKS:							
DRINKS:							
TOTAL							

WATER (8-oz glasses OR 2 litres of water a day):		Yes ✕	No ✕

TOTAL SLEEP / REST HOURS	NIGHT	DAY	TOTAL

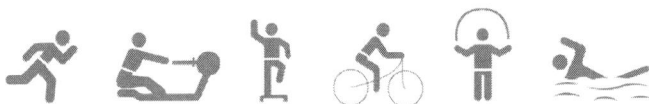

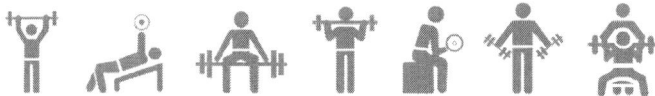

Day/Date: _____   Time/Duration: _____

WEIGHT TRAINING

Muscle Group(s)   **Chest**   **Shoulders**   **Back**   **Arms**   **Legs**   **Abs**

| EXERCISE | Set 1 | | Set 2 | | Set 3 | | Set 4 | | Rest between Sets | Set 5 or the Set with Max. Wt./Reps | |
	Weight	Reps	Weight	Reps	Weight	Reps	Weight	Reps		Weight	Reps

CARDIO & STRETCHING   Time/Duration: _____   **NOTES**

| EXERCISE / LEVEL | Time/ Duration | | Distance | | Calories | | Ideas/goals for next session: |
	Goal	Actual	Goal	Actual	Goal	Actual	

DIET & SLEEP

MEALS	Protein	Carbs	Total Fat	Sugars	Sodium/ Salt	Fiber	Calories
BREAKFAST:							
LUNCH:							
DINNER:							
SNACKS:							
DRINKS:							
TOTAL							

WATER (8-oz glasses OR 2 litres of water a day):		Yes ✕	No ✕

TOTAL SLEEP / REST HOURS	**NIGHT**	**DAY**	**TOTAL**

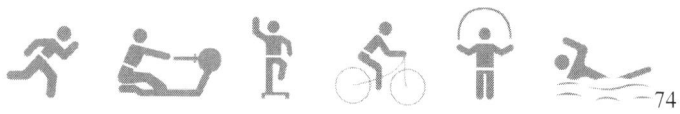

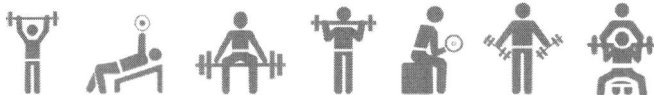

WEIGHT TRAINING

Day/Date: Time/Duration:

Muscle Group(s)	Chest		Shoulders		Back		Arms			Legs	Abs
	Set 1		Set 2		Set 3		Set 4		Rest between Sets	Set 5 or the Set with Max. Wt./Reps	
EXERCISE	Weight	Reps	Weight	Reps	Weight	Reps	Weight	Reps		Weight	Reps

CARDIO & STRETCHING   Time/Duration: NOTES

EXERCISE / LEVEL	Time/ Duration		Distance		Calories		Ideas/goals for next session:
	Goal	Actual	Goal	Actual	Goal	Actual	

DIET & SLEEP

MEALS	Protein	Carbs	Total Fat	Sugars	Sodium/ Salt	Fiber	Calories
BREAKFAST:							
LUNCH:							
DINNER:							
SNACKS:							
DRINKS:							
TOTAL							

WATER (8-oz glasses OR 2 litres of water a day):		Yes	╳	No	╳

TOTAL SLEEP / REST HOURS	NIGHT	DAY	TOTAL

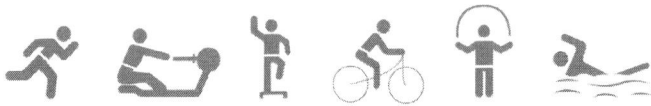

Day/Date: **Time/Duration:**

WEIGHT TRAINING

Muscle Group(s) Chest   Shoulders   Back   Arms   Legs   Abs

EXERCISE	Set 1 Weight	Set 1 Reps	Set 2 Weight	Set 2 Reps	Set 3 Weight	Set 3 Reps	Set 4 Weight	Set 4 Reps	Rest between Sets	Set 5 or the Set with Max. Wt./Reps Weight	Reps

CARDIO & STRETCHING   Time/Duration: NOTES

Ideas/goals for next session:

EXERCISE / LEVEL	Time/Duration Goal	Time/Duration Actual	Distance Goal	Distance Actual	Calories Goal	Calories Actual

DIET & SLEEP

MEALS	Protein	Carbs	Total Fat	Sugars	Sodium/Salt	Fiber	Calories
BREAKFAST:							
LUNCH:							
DINNER:							
SNACKS:							
DRINKS:							
TOTAL							

WATER (8-oz glasses OR 2 litres of water a day):   Yes   ✕   No   ✕

TOTAL SLEEP / REST HOURS	NIGHT	DAY	TOTAL

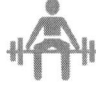

Day/Date: _____   Time/Duration: _____

WEIGHT TRAINING

Muscle Group(s)   Chest   Shoulders   Back   Arms   Legs   Abs

EXERCISE	Set 1 Weight	Set 1 Reps	Set 2 Weight	Set 2 Reps	Set 3 Weight	Set 3 Reps	Set 4 Weight	Set 4 Reps	Rest between Sets	Set 5 or the Set with Max. Wt./Reps Weight	Reps

CARDIO & STRETCHING   Time/Duration: _____   NOTES

Ideas/goals for next session:

EXERCISE / LEVEL	Time/Duration Goal	Actual	Distance Goal	Actual	Calories Goal	Actual

DIET & SLEEP

MEALS	Protein	Carbs	Total Fat	Sugars	Sodium/Salt	Fiber	Calories
BREAKFAST:							
LUNCH:							
DINNER:							
SNACKS:							
DRINKS:							
TOTAL							

WATER (8-oz glasses OR 2 litres of water a day):	Yes ✕	No ✕

TOTAL SLEEP / REST HOURS	NIGHT	DAY	TOTAL

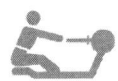 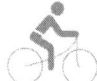

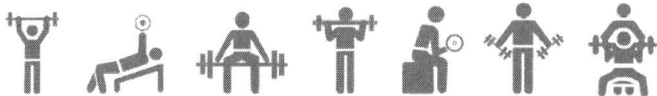

WEIGHT TRAINING

Day/Date: _____   Time/Duration: _____

Muscle Group(s)	Chest		Shoulders		Back		Arms		Rest between Sets	Legs	Abs
	Set 1		Set 2		Set 3		Set 4			Set 5 or the Set with Max. Wt./Reps	
EXERCISE	Weight	Reps	Weight	Reps	Weight	Reps	Weight	Reps		Weight	Reps

CARDIO & STRETCHING   Time/Duration: _____   NOTES

Ideas/goals for next session:

EXERCISE / LEVEL	Time/ Duration		Distance		Calories	
	Goal	Actual	Goal	Actual	Goal	Actual

DIET & SLEEP

MEALS	Protein	Carbs	Total Fat	Sugars	Sodium/ Salt	Fiber	Calories
BREAKFAST:							
LUNCH:							
DINNER:							
SNACKS:							
DRINKS:							
TOTAL							

WATER (8-oz glasses OR 2 litres of water a day):   Yes ✕   No ✕

TOTAL SLEEP / REST HOURS	NIGHT	DAY	TOTAL

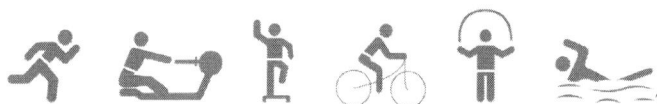

78

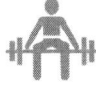

Day/Date: _____   Time/Duration: _____

WEIGHT TRAINING

Muscle Group(s) **Chest   Shoulders   Back   Arms   Legs   Abs**

EXERCISE	Set 1		Set 2		Set 3		Set 4		Rest between Sets	Set 5 or the Set with Max. Wt./Reps	
	Weight	Reps	Weight	Reps	Weight	Reps	Weight	Reps		Weight	Reps

CARDIO & STRETCHING   Time/Duration: _____   *NOTES*

EXERCISE / LEVEL	Time/ Duration		Distance		Calories		Ideas/goals for next session:
	Goal	Actual	Goal	Actual	Goal	Actual	

DIET & SLEEP

MEALS	Protein	Carbs	Total Fat	Sugars	Sodium/ Salt	Fiber	Calories
BREAKFAST:							
LUNCH:							
DINNER:							
SNACKS:							
DRINKS:							
TOTAL							

WATER (8-oz glasses OR 2 litres of water a day):   Yes   ✕   No   ✕

TOTAL SLEEP / REST HOURS	NIGHT	DAY	TOTAL

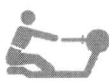 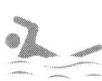

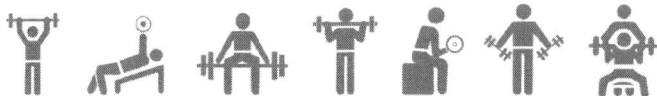

Day/Date: _____   Time/Duration: _____

WEIGHT TRAINING

Muscle Group(s)   Chest   Shoulders   Back   Arms   Legs   Abs

EXERCISE	Set 1 Weight	Set 1 Reps	Set 2 Weight	Set 2 Reps	Set 3 Weight	Set 3 Reps	Set 4 Weight	Set 4 Reps	Rest between Sets	Set 5 or the Set with Max. Wt./Reps Weight	Reps

CARDIO & STRETCHING   Time/Duration: _____   NOTES

EXERCISE / LEVEL	Time/Duration Goal	Actual	Distance Goal	Actual	Calories Goal	Actual

Ideas/goals for next session:

DIET & SLEEP

MEALS	Protein	Carbs	Total Fat	Sugars	Sodium/Salt	Fiber	Calories
BREAKFAST:							
LUNCH:							
DINNER:							
SNACKS:							
DRINKS:							
TOTAL							

WATER (8-oz glasses OR 2 litres of water a day):   Yes   ×   No   ×

TOTAL SLEEP / REST HOURS	NIGHT	DAY	TOTAL

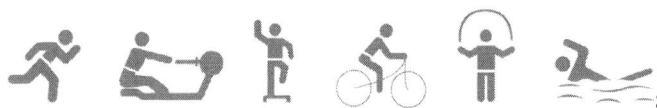

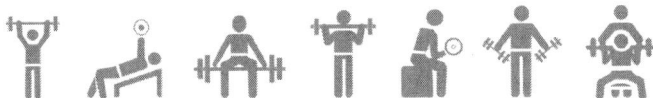

WEIGHT TRAINING

Day/Date: _____   Time/Duration: _____

Muscle Group(s)	Chest		Shoulders		Back		Arms		Rest between Sets	Legs Abs — Set 5 or the Set with Max. Wt./Reps	
EXERCISE	Set 1		Set 2		Set 3		Set 4				
	Weight	Reps	Weight	Reps	Weight	Reps	Weight	Reps		Weight	Reps

CARDIO & STRETCHING   Time/Duration: _____   NOTES

Ideas/goals for next session:

EXERCISE / LEVEL	Time/ Duration		Distance		Calories	
	Goal	Actual	Goal	Actual	Goal	Actual

DIET & SLEEP

MEALS	Protein	Carbs	Total Fat	Sugars	Sodium/ Salt	Fiber	Calories
BREAKFAST:							
LUNCH:							
DINNER:							
SNACKS:							
DRINKS:							
TOTAL							

WATER (8-oz glasses OR 2 litres of water a day):   Yes ✕   No ✕

TOTAL SLEEP / REST HOURS	NIGHT	DAY	TOTAL

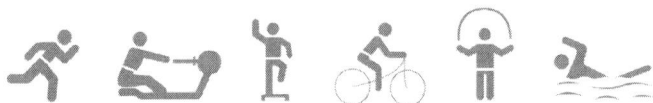

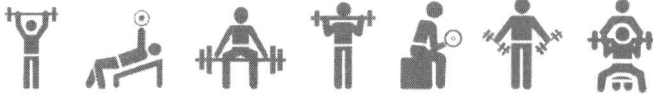

Day/Date: _____   Time/Duration: _____

WEIGHT TRAINING

Muscle Group(s) Chest   Shoulders   Back   Arms   Legs   Abs

EXERCISE	Set 1 Weight	Set 1 Reps	Set 2 Weight	Set 2 Reps	Set 3 Weight	Set 3 Reps	Set 4 Weight	Set 4 Reps	Rest between Sets	Set 5 or the Set with Max. Wt./Reps Weight	Reps

CARDIO & STRETCHING   Time/Duration: _____   NOTES

Ideas/goals for next session:

EXERCISE / LEVEL	Time/Duration Goal	Time/Duration Actual	Distance Goal	Distance Actual	Calories Goal	Calories Actual

DIET & SLEEP

MEALS	Protein	Carbs	Total Fat	Sugars	Sodium/Salt	Fiber	Calories
BREAKFAST:							
LUNCH:							
DINNER:							
SNACKS:							
DRINKS:							
TOTAL							

WATER (8-oz glasses OR 2 litres of water a day):   Yes ✕   No ✕

TOTAL SLEEP / REST HOURS	NIGHT	DAY	TOTAL

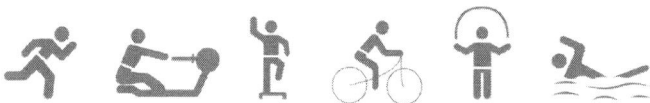

82

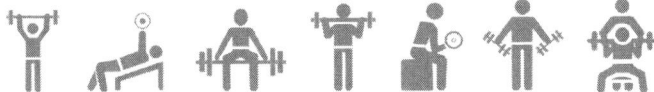

WEIGHT TRAINING   Day/Date: _____   Time/Duration: _____

Muscle Group(s)	Chest		Shoulders		Back		Arms		Rest between Sets	Legs Abs Set 5 or the Set with Max. Wt./Reps	
	Set 1		Set 2		Set 3		Set 4				
EXERCISE	Weight	Reps	Weight	Reps	Weight	Reps	Weight	Reps		Weight	Reps

CARDIO & STRETCHING   Time/Duration: _____

EXERCISE / LEVEL	Time/ Duration		Distance		Calories		NOTES — Ideas/goals for next session:
	Goal	Actual	Goal	Actual	Goal	Actual	

DIET & SLEEP

MEALS	Protein	Carbs	Total Fat	Sugars	Sodium/Salt	Fiber	Calories
BREAKFAST:							
LUNCH:							
DINNER:							
SNACKS:							
DRINKS:							
TOTAL							

WATER (8-oz glasses OR 2 litres of water a day):	Yes ✗	No ✗

TOTAL SLEEP / REST HOURS	NIGHT	DAY	TOTAL

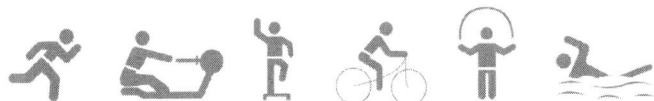

83

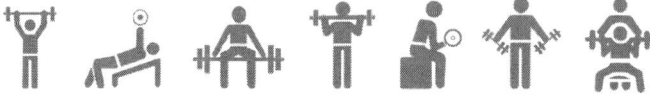

	Day/Date:						Time/Duration:		

WEIGHT TRAINING

Muscle Group(s)   **Chest**   **Shoulders**   **Back**   **Arms**   **Legs**   **Abs**

EXERCISE	Set 1		Set 2		Set 3		Set 4		Rest between Sets	Set 5 or the Set with Max. Wt./Reps	
	Weight	Reps	Weight	Reps	Weight	Reps	Weight	Reps		Weight	Reps

CARDIO & STRETCHING   Time/Duration: NOTES

EXERCISE / LEVEL	Time/ Duration		Distance		Calories		Ideas/goals for next session:
	Goal	Actual	Goal	Actual	Goal	Actual	

DIET & SLEEP

MEALS	Protein	Carbs	Total Fat	Sugars	Sodium/ Salt	Fiber	Calories
BREAKFAST:							
LUNCH:							
DINNER:							
SNACKS:							
DRINKS:							
TOTAL							

WATER (8-oz glasses OR 2 litres of water a day):		Yes ✕	No ✕

TOTAL SLEEP / REST HOURS	NIGHT	DAY	TOTAL

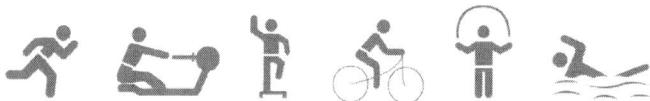

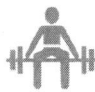

| | Day/Date: | | | Time/Duration: | |

WEIGHT TRAINING

Muscle Group(s) Chest   Shoulders   Back   Arms   Legs   Abs

| EXERCISE | Set 1 | | Set 2 | | Set 3 | | Set 4 | | Rest between Sets | Set 5 or the Set with Max. Wt./Reps | |
	Weight	Reps	Weight	Reps	Weight	Reps	Weight	Reps		Weight	Reps

CARDIO & STRETCHING   Time/Duration: *NOTES*

Ideas/goals for next session:

| EXERCISE / LEVEL | Time/ Duration | | Distance | | Calories | |
	Goal	Actual	Goal	Actual	Goal	Actual

DIET & SLEEP

MEALS	Protein	Carbs	Total Fat	Sugars	Sodium/ Salt	Fiber	Calories
BREAKFAST:							
LUNCH:							
DINNER:							
SNACKS:							
DRINKS:							
TOTAL							

WATER (8-oz glasses OR 2 litres of water a day):   Yes   ✕   No   ✕

TOTAL SLEEP / REST HOURS	NIGHT	DAY	TOTAL

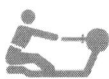 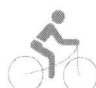

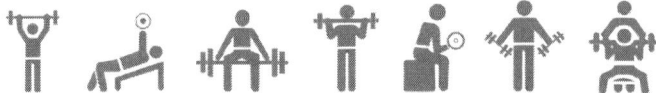

Day/Date: **Time/Duration:**

WEIGHT TRAINING

Muscle Group(s)   Chest   Shoulders   Back   Arms   Legs   Abs

EXERCISE	Set 1 Weight	Set 1 Reps	Set 2 Weight	Set 2 Reps	Set 3 Weight	Set 3 Reps	Set 4 Weight	Set 4 Reps	Rest between Sets	Set 5 or the Set with Max. Wt./Reps Weight	Reps

CARDIO & STRETCHING   Time/Duration: NOTES

Ideas/goals for next session:

EXERCISE / LEVEL	Time/Duration Goal	Time/Duration Actual	Distance Goal	Distance Actual	Calories Goal	Calories Actual

DIET & SLEEP

MEALS	Protein	Carbs	Total Fat	Sugars	Sodium/Salt	Fiber	Calories
BREAKFAST:							
LUNCH:							
DINNER:							
SNACKS:							
DRINKS:							
TOTAL							

WATER (8-oz glasses OR 2 litres of water a day):   Yes   ×   No   ×

TOTAL SLEEP / REST HOURS	NIGHT	DAY	TOTAL

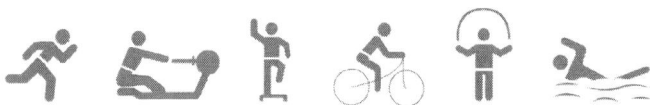

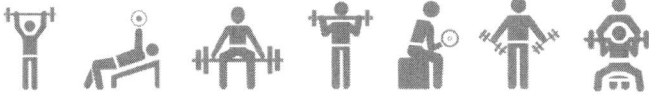

Day/Date: _____   Time/Duration: _____

WEIGHT TRAINING

Muscle Group(s)   **Chest   Shoulders   Back   Arms   Legs   Abs**

EXERCISE	Set 1 Weight	Set 1 Reps	Set 2 Weight	Set 2 Reps	Set 3 Weight	Set 3 Reps	Set 4 Weight	Set 4 Reps	Rest between Sets	Set 5 or the Set with Max. Wt./Reps Weight	Reps

CARDIO & STRETCHING   Time/Duration: _____   NOTES

EXERCISE / LEVEL	Time/Duration Goal	Actual	Distance Goal	Actual	Calories Goal	Actual	Ideas/goals for next session:

DIET & SLEEP

MEALS	Protein	Carbs	Total Fat	Sugars	Sodium/Salt	Fiber	Calories
BREAKFAST:							
LUNCH:							
DINNER:							
SNACKS:							
DRINKS:							
TOTAL							

WATER (8-oz glasses OR 2 litres of water a day):	Yes ✗	No ✗

TOTAL SLEEP / REST HOURS	NIGHT	DAY	TOTAL

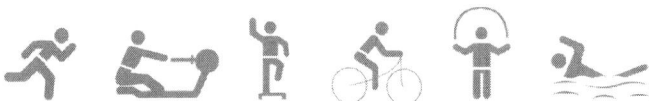

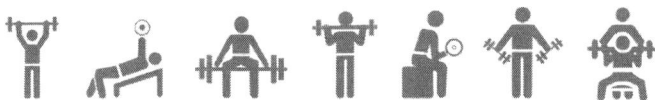

Day/Date: _____   **Time/Duration:** _____

WEIGHT TRAINING

Muscle Group(s)   **Chest**   **Shoulders**   **Back**   **Arms**   **Legs**   **Abs**

EXERCISE	Set 1 Weight	Set 1 Reps	Set 2 Weight	Set 2 Reps	Set 3 Weight	Set 3 Reps	Set 4 Weight	Set 4 Reps	Rest between Sets	Set 5 or the Set with Max. Wt./Reps Weight	Reps

CARDIO & STRETCHING   **Time/Duration:** _____   NOTES

Ideas/goals for next session:

EXERCISE / LEVEL	Time/Duration Goal	Actual	Distance Goal	Actual	Calories Goal	Actual

DIET & SLEEP

MEALS	Protein	Carbs	Total Fat	Sugars	Sodium/Salt	Fiber	Calories
BREAKFAST:							
LUNCH:							
DINNER:							
SNACKS:							
DRINKS:							
TOTAL							

WATER (8-oz glasses OR 2 litres of water a day):		Yes ✕	No ✕

TOTAL SLEEP / REST HOURS	**NIGHT**	**DAY**	**TOTAL**

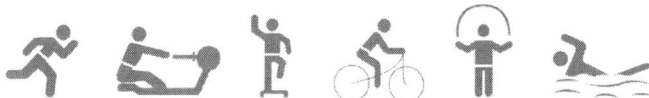

Day/Date: _____   Time/Duration: _____

WEIGHT TRAINING

Muscle Group(s)	Chest		Shoulders		Back		Arms		Rest between Sets	Legs Abs Set 5 or the Set with Max. Wt./Reps	
EXERCISE	Set 1		Set 2		Set 3		Set 4				
	Weight	Reps	Weight	Reps	Weight	Reps	Weight	Reps		Weight	Reps

CARDIO & STRETCHING   Time/Duration: _____

NOTES

Ideas/goals for next session:

EXERCISE / LEVEL	Time/ Duration		Distance		Calories	
	Goal	Actual	Goal	Actual	Goal	Actual

DIET & SLEEP

MEALS	Protein	Carbs	Total Fat	Sugars	Sodium/ Salt	Fiber	Calories
BREAKFAST:							
LUNCH:							
DINNER:							
SNACKS:							
DRINKS:							
TOTAL							

WATER (8-oz glasses OR 2 litres of water a day):		Yes ✕	No ✕	
TOTAL SLEEP / REST HOURS	**NIGHT**	**DAY**	**TOTAL**	

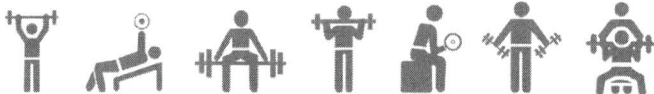

WEIGHT TRAINING

Day/Date: Time/Duration:

Muscle Group(s)   Chest   Shoulders   Back   Arms   Legs   Abs

EXERCISE	Set 1 Weight	Set 1 Reps	Set 2 Weight	Set 2 Reps	Set 3 Weight	Set 3 Reps	Set 4 Weight	Set 4 Reps	Rest between Sets	Set 5 or the Set with Max. Wt./Reps Weight	Set 5 or the Set with Max. Wt./Reps Reps

CARDIO & STRETCHING   Time/Duration: NOTES

EXERCISE / LEVEL	Time/ Duration Goal	Time/ Duration Actual	Distance Goal	Distance Actual	Calories Goal	Calories Actual	Ideas/goals for next session:

DIET & SLEEP

MEALS	Protein	Carbs	Total Fat	Sugars	Sodium/ Salt	Fiber	Calories
BREAKFAST:							
LUNCH:							
DINNER:							
SNACKS:							
DRINKS:							
TOTAL							

WATER (8-oz glasses OR 2 litres of water a day):   Yes ✕ No ✕

TOTAL SLEEP / REST HOURS	NIGHT	DAY	TOTAL

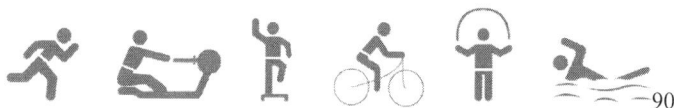

WEIGHT TRAINING

Day/Date: Time/Duration:

Muscle Group(s)   Chest   Shoulders   Back   Arms   Legs   Abs

EXERCISE	Set 1 Weight	Set 1 Reps	Set 2 Weight	Set 2 Reps	Set 3 Weight	Set 3 Reps	Set 4 Weight	Set 4 Reps	Rest between Sets	Set 5 or the Set with Max. Wt./Reps Weight	Reps

CARDIO & STRETCHING

Time/Duration: *NOTES*

EXERCISE / LEVEL	Time/ Duration Goal	Actual	Distance Goal	Actual	Calories Goal	Actual

Ideas/goals for next session:

DIET & SLEEP

MEALS	Protein	Carbs	Total Fat	Sugars	Sodium/ Salt	Fiber	Calories
BREAKFAST:							
LUNCH:							
DINNER:							
SNACKS:							
DRINKS:							
TOTAL							

WATER (8-oz glasses OR 2 litres of water a day):   Yes   No

TOTAL SLEEP / REST HOURS	NIGHT	DAY	TOTAL

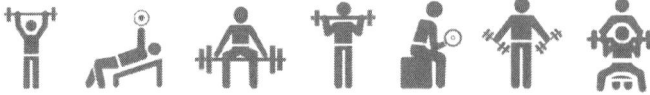

WEIGHT TRAINING

Day/Date: _____   Time/Duration: _____

Muscle Group(s)	Chest		Shoulders		Back		Arms		Rest between Sets	Legs	Abs
	Set 1		Set 2		Set 3		Set 4			Set 5 or the Set with Max. Wt./Reps	
EXERCISE	Weight	Reps	Weight	Reps	Weight	Reps	Weight	Reps		Weight	Reps

CARDIO & STRETCHING   Time/Duration: _____   NOTES

EXERCISE / LEVEL	Time/Duration		Distance		Calories		Ideas/goals for next session:
	Goal	Actual	Goal	Actual	Goal	Actual	

DIET & SLEEP

MEALS	Protein	Carbs	Total Fat	Sugars	Sodium/Salt	Fiber	Calories
BREAKFAST:							
LUNCH:							
DINNER:							
SNACKS:							
DRINKS:							
TOTAL							
WATER (8-oz glasses OR 2 litres of water a day):				Yes ✕		No ✕	

TOTAL SLEEP / REST HOURS	NIGHT	DAY	TOTAL

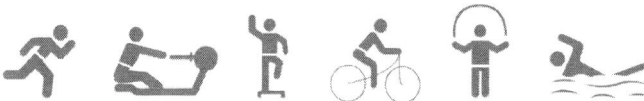

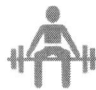

Day/Date: _____ *Time/Duration:* _____

WEIGHT TRAINING

Muscle Group(s)   **Chest**   **Shoulders**   **Back**   **Arms**   **Legs**   **Abs**

EXERCISE	Set 1		Set 2		Set 3		Set 4		Rest between Sets	Set 5 or the Set with Max. Wt./Reps	
	Weight	Reps	Weight	Reps	Weight	Reps	Weight	Reps		Weight	Reps

CARDIO & STRETCHING   Time/Duration: _____   *NOTES*

EXERCISE / LEVEL	Time/ Duration		Distance		Calories		Ideas/goals for next session:
	Goal	Actual	Goal	Actual	Goal	Actual	

DIET & SLEEP

MEALS	Protein	Carbs	Total Fat	Sugars	Sodium/ Salt	Fiber	Calories
BREAKFAST:							
LUNCH:							
DINNER:							
SNACKS:							
DRINKS:							
TOTAL							

WATER (8-oz glasses OR 2 litres of water a day):   Yes   No

TOTAL SLEEP / REST HOURS	**NIGHT**	**DAY**	**TOTAL**

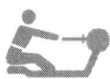 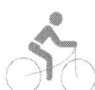 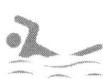

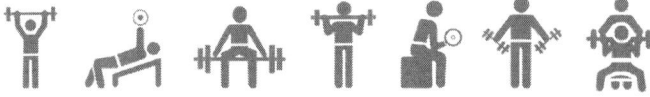

Day/Date: _____   Time/Duration: _____

WEIGHT TRAINING

Muscle Group(s)   Chest   Shoulders   Back   Arms   Legs   Abs

EXERCISE	Set 1		Set 2		Set 3		Set 4		Rest between Sets	Set 5 or the Set with Max. Wt./Reps	
	Weight	Reps	Weight	Reps	Weight	Reps	Weight	Reps		Weight	Reps

CARDIO & STRETCHING   Time/Duration: _____

NOTES
Ideas/goals for next session:

EXERCISE / LEVEL	Time/Duration		Distance		Calories	
	Goal	Actual	Goal	Actual	Goal	Actual

DIET & SLEEP

MEALS	Protein	Carbs	Total Fat	Sugars	Sodium/Salt	Fiber	Calories
BREAKFAST:							
LUNCH:							
DINNER:							
SNACKS:							
DRINKS:							
TOTAL							

WATER (8-oz glasses OR 2 litres of water a day):	Yes ✕	No ✕

TOTAL SLEEP / REST HOURS	NIGHT	DAY	TOTAL

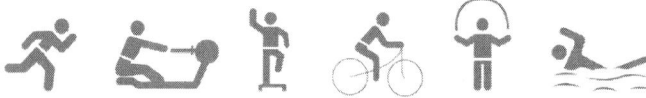

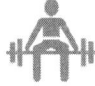

Day/Date: _____   Time/Duration: _____

WEIGHT TRAINING

Muscle Group(s)   **Chest   Shoulders   Back   Arms   Legs   Abs**

EXERCISE	Set 1		Set 2		Set 3		Set 4		Rest between Sets	Set 5 or the Set with Max. Wt./Reps	
	Weight	Reps	Weight	Reps	Weight	Reps	Weight	Reps		Weight	Reps

CARDIO & STRETCHING   Time/Duration: _____   NOTES

EXERCISE / LEVEL	Time/ Duration		Distance		Calories	
	Goal	Actual	Goal	Actual	Goal	Actual

Ideas/goals for next session:

DIET & SLEEP

MEALS	Protein	Carbs	Total Fat	Sugars	Sodium/ Salt	Fiber	Calories
BREAKFAST:							
LUNCH:							
DINNER:							
SNACKS:							
DRINKS:							
TOTAL							

WATER (8-oz glasses OR 2 litres of water a day):	Yes	No

TOTAL SLEEP / REST HOURS	NIGHT	DAY	TOTAL

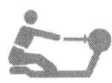
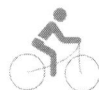

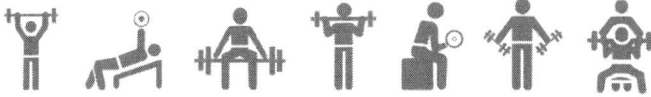

WEIGHT TRAINING

Day/Date: Time/Duration:

Muscle Group(s)	Chest		Shoulders		Back		Arms		Rest between Sets	Legs Abs Set 5 or the Set with Max. Wt./Reps	
EXERCISE	Set 1		Set 2		Set 3		Set 4				
	Weight	Reps	Weight	Reps	Weight	Reps	Weight	Reps		Weight	Reps

CARDIO & STRETCHING

Time/Duration: **NOTES**

Ideas/goals for next session:

EXERCISE / LEVEL	Time/ Duration		Distance		Calories	
	Goal	Actual	Goal	Actual	Goal	Actual

DIET & SLEEP

MEALS	Protein	Carbs	Total Fat	Sugars	Sodium/ Salt	Fiber	Calories
BREAKFAST:							
LUNCH:							
DINNER:							
SNACKS:							
DRINKS:							
TOTAL							
WATER (8-oz glasses OR 2 litres of water a day):					Yes ×	No ×	

TOTAL SLEEP / REST HOURS	NIGHT	DAY	TOTAL

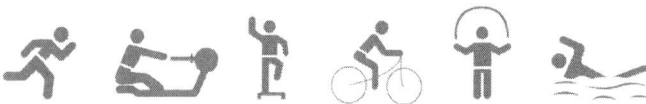

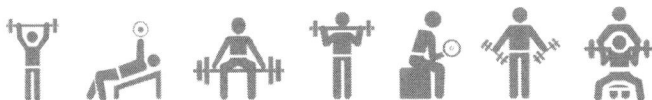

WEIGHT TRAINING

Day/Date: Time/Duration:

Muscle Group(s)	Chest		Shoulders		Back		Arms		Rest between Sets	Legs	Abs
	Set 1		Set 2		Set 3		Set 4			Set 5 or the Set with Max. Wt./Reps	
EXERCISE	Weight	Reps	Weight	Reps	Weight	Reps	Weight	Reps		Weight	Reps

CARDIO & STRETCHING   Time/Duration: NOTES

EXERCISE / LEVEL	Time/ Duration		Distance		Calories		Ideas/goals for next session:
	Goal	Actual	Goal	Actual	Goal	Actual	

DIET & SLEEP

MEALS	Protein	Carbs	Total Fat	Sugars	Sodium/ Salt	Fiber	Calories
BREAKFAST:							
LUNCH:							
DINNER:							
SNACKS:							
DRINKS:							
TOTAL							

WATER (8-oz glasses OR 2 litres of water a day):   Yes   No

TOTAL SLEEP / REST HOURS	NIGHT	DAY	TOTAL

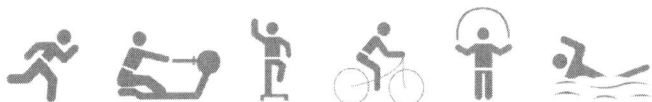

97

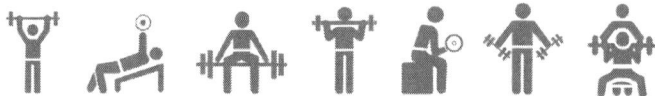

Day/Date: _____   Time/Duration: _____

WEIGHT TRAINING

Muscle Group(s)	Chest		Shoulders		Back		Arms		Rest between Sets	Legs Abs	
	Set 1		Set 2		Set 3		Set 4			Set 5 or the Set with Max. Wt./Reps	
EXERCISE	Weight	Reps	Weight	Reps	Weight	Reps	Weight	Reps		Weight	Reps

CARDIO & STRETCHING   Time/Duration: _____   NOTES

EXERCISE / LEVEL	Time/ Duration		Distance		Calories		Ideas/goals for next session:
	Goal	Actual	Goal	Actual	Goal	Actual	

DIET & SLEEP

MEALS	Protein	Carbs	Total Fat	Sugars	Sodium/ Salt	Fiber	Calories
BREAKFAST:							
LUNCH:							
DINNER:							
SNACKS:							
DRINKS:							
TOTAL							
WATER (8-oz glasses OR 2 litres of water a day):					Yes ☒	No	☒

TOTAL SLEEP / REST HOURS	NIGHT	DAY	TOTAL

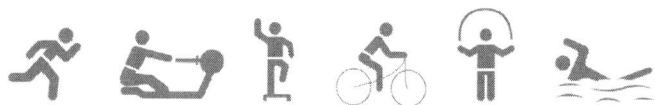

WEIGHT TRAINING

Day/Date: Time/Duration:

Muscle Group(s)	Chest		Shoulders		Back		Arms		Rest between Sets	Legs Abs — Set 5 or the Set with Max. Wt./Reps	
	Set 1		Set 2		Set 3		Set 4				
EXERCISE	Weight	Reps	Weight	Reps	Weight	Reps	Weight	Reps		Weight	Reps

CARDIO & STRETCHING   Time/Duration: NOTES

EXERCISE / LEVEL	Time/ Duration		Distance		Calories		Ideas/goals for next session:
	Goal	Actual	Goal	Actual	Goal	Actual	

DIET & SLEEP

MEALS	Protein	Carbs	Total Fat	Sugars	Sodium/ Salt	Fiber	Calories
BREAKFAST:							
LUNCH:							
DINNER:							
SNACKS:							
DRINKS:							
TOTAL							

WATER (8-oz glasses OR 2 litres of water a day):   Yes   ✕   No   ✕

TOTAL SLEEP / REST HOURS	NIGHT	DAY	TOTAL

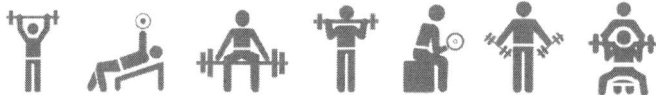

Day/Date: _____ **Time/Duration:** _____

WEIGHT TRAINING

Muscle Group(s)   Chest   Shoulders   Back   Arms   Legs   Abs

EXERCISE	Set 1		Set 2		Set 3		Set 4		Rest between Sets	Set 5 or the Set with Max. Wt./Reps	
	Weight	Reps	Weight	Reps	Weight	Reps	Weight	Reps		Weight	Reps

CARDIO & STRETCHING   Time/Duration: _____   NOTES

Ideas/goals for next session:

EXERCISE / LEVEL	Time/Duration		Distance		Calories	
	Goal	Actual	Goal	Actual	Goal	Actual

DIET & SLEEP

MEALS	Protein	Carbs	Total Fat	Sugars	Sodium/Salt	Fiber	Calories
BREAKFAST:							
LUNCH:							
DINNER:							
SNACKS:							
DRINKS:							
TOTAL							

WATER (8-oz glasses OR 2 litres of water a day):   Yes ✕   No ✕

TOTAL SLEEP / REST HOURS	NIGHT	DAY	TOTAL

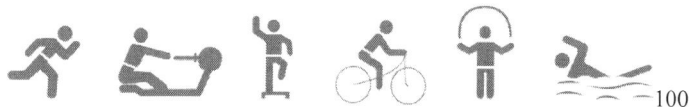

Day/Date: _____ *Time/Duration:* _____

WEIGHT TRAINING

Muscle Group(s) **Chest** **Shoulders** **Back** **Arms** **Legs Abs**

EXERCISE	Set 1		Set 2		Set 3		Set 4		Rest between Sets	Set 5 or the Set with Max. Wt./Reps	
	Weight	Reps	Weight	Reps	Weight	Reps	Weight	Reps		Weight	Reps

CARDIO & STRETCHING   Time/Duration: NOTES

EXERCISE / LEVEL	Time/ Duration		Distance		Calories		Ideas/goals for next session:
	Goal	Actual	Goal	Actual	Goal	Actual	

DIET & SLEEP

MEALS	Protein	Carbs	Total Fat	Sugars	Sodium/ Salt	Fiber	Calories
BREAKFAST:							
LUNCH:							
DINNER:							
SNACKS:							
DRINKS:							
TOTAL							

WATER (8-oz glasses OR 2 litres of water a day):	Yes	No

	NIGHT	DAY	TOTAL
TOTAL SLEEP / REST HOURS			

101

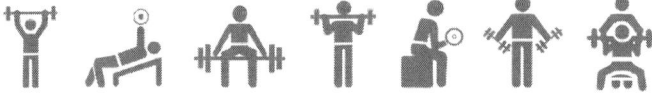

WEIGHT TRAINING

Day/Date: _____   Time/Duration: _____

| Muscle Group(s) | Chest | Shoulders | Back | Arms | Legs | Abs |

EXERCISE	Set 1 Weight	Reps	Set 2 Weight	Reps	Set 3 Weight	Reps	Set 4 Weight	Reps	Rest between Sets	Set 5 or the Set with Max. Wt./Reps Weight	Reps

CARDIO & STRETCHING   Time/Duration: _____

NOTES
Ideas/goals for next session:

EXERCISE / LEVEL	Time/ Duration Goal	Actual	Distance Goal	Actual	Calories Goal	Actual

DIET & SLEEP

MEALS	Protein	Carbs	Total Fat	Sugars	Sodium/ Salt	Fiber	Calories
BREAKFAST:							
LUNCH:							
DINNER:							
SNACKS:							
DRINKS:							
TOTAL							

WATER (8-oz glasses OR 2 litres of water a day):   Yes ×   No ×

TOTAL SLEEP / REST HOURS	NIGHT	DAY	TOTAL

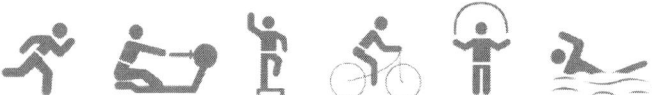

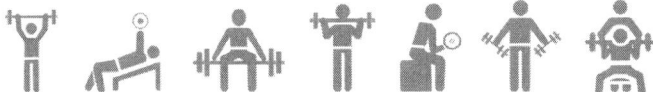

Day/Date: Time/Duration:

WEIGHT TRAINING

Muscle Group(s)	Chest		Shoulders		Back		Arms		Rest between Sets	Set 5 or the Set with Max. Wt./Reps	
	Set 1		Set 2		Set 3		Set 4			Legs	Abs
EXERCISE	Weight	Reps	Weight	Reps	Weight	Reps	Weight	Reps		Weight	Reps

CARDIO & STRETCHING   Time/Duration: NOTES

EXERCISE / LEVEL	Time/Duration		Distance		Calories		Ideas/goals for next session:
	Goal	Actual	Goal	Actual	Goal	Actual	

DIET & SLEEP

MEALS	Protein	Carbs	Total Fat	Sugars	Sodium/Salt	Fiber	Calories
BREAKFAST:							
LUNCH:							
DINNER:							
SNACKS:							
DRINKS:							
TOTAL							

WATER (8-oz glasses OR 2 litres of water a day):   Yes   ✕   No   ✕

TOTAL SLEEP / REST HOURS	NIGHT	DAY	TOTAL

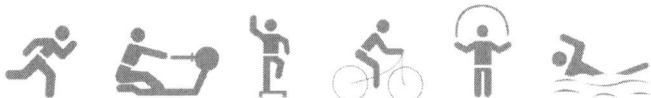

	Day/Date:						Time/Duration:				

WEIGHT TRAINING

Muscle Group(s)	Chest		Shoulders		Back		Arms		Rest between Sets	Set 5 or the Set with Max. Wt./Reps	
	Set 1		Set 2		Set 3		Set 4			Legs	Abs
EXERCISE	Weight	Reps	Weight	Reps	Weight	Reps	Weight	Reps		Weight	Reps

CARDIO & STRETCHING			Time/Duration:				NOTES

	Time/ Duration		Distance		Calories		Ideas/goals for next session:
EXERCISE / LEVEL	Goal	Actual	Goal	Actual	Goal	Actual	

DIET & SLEEP

MEALS	Protein	Carbs	Total Fat	Sugars	Sodium/Salt	Fiber	Calories
BREAKFAST:							
LUNCH:							
DINNER:							
SNACKS:							
DRINKS:							
TOTAL							
WATER (8-oz glasses OR 2 litres of water a day):					Yes ✕	No ✕	

	NIGHT	DAY	TOTAL
TOTAL SLEEP / REST HOURS			

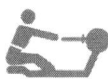 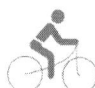 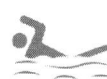

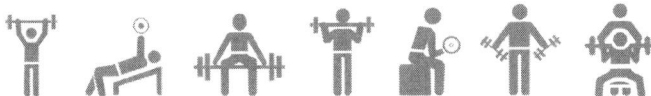

WEIGHT TRAINING

Day/Date:　　　　Time/Duration:

Muscle Group(s)	Chest		Shoulders		Back		Arms		Rest between Sets	Set 5 or the Set with Max. Wt./Reps	
EXERCISE	Set 1		Set 2		Set 3		Set 4				
	Weight	Reps	Weight	Reps	Weight	Reps	Weight	Reps		Weight	Reps

CARDIO & STRETCHING　　　Time/Duration:　　　　NOTES

EXERCISE / LEVEL	Time/ Duration		Distance		Calories		Ideas/goals for next session:
	Goal	Actual	Goal	Actual	Goal	Actual	

DIET & SLEEP

MEALS	Protein	Carbs	Total Fat	Sugars	Sodium/ Salt	Fiber	Calories
BREAKFAST:							
LUNCH:							
DINNER:							
SNACKS:							
DRINKS:							
TOTAL							

WATER (8-oz glasses OR 2 litres of water a day):		Yes	×	No	×
TOTAL SLEEP / REST HOURS	**NIGHT**	**DAY**		**TOTAL**	

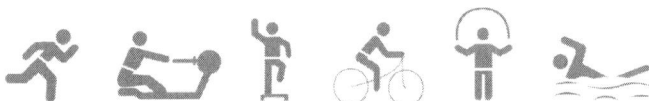

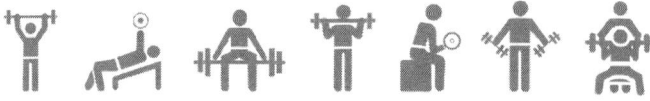

Weekly Review and Planning

Feeling fitter today… bring on next week!

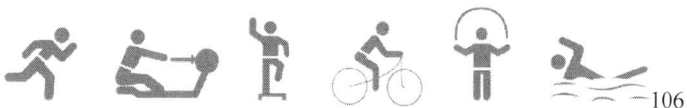

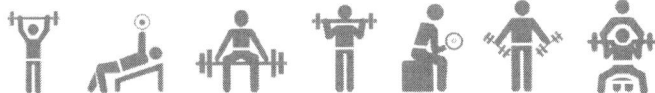

WEEKLY REVIEW Week of : *July 2-8, 2018*

EXERCISE	Number of sessions	Mon	Tue	Wed	Thu	Fri	Sat	Sun
Weight Training	4	×	×		×	×		
Cardio	3			×			×	×
Stretching	5	×	×	×	×	×		

Muscle Group(s)	Number of sessions	Mon	Tue	Wed	Thu	Fri	Sat	Sun
Chest	2	×		×	×			
Shoulders	1					×		
Back	2		×			×		
Arms	2	×			×			
Legs	1		×					
Abs	3			×			×	×

Weekly training target(s) achieved?					Yes		No	
Great week, completed all planned sessions					×			

Did I sleep for 56 hrs in the week?		Mon	Tue	Wed	Thu	Fri	Sat	Sun
Total Sleep Hours	56	7.5	7.5	8	7.5	8	9	8.5

Notes:

Highlight/achievement of the week:

Increased bench press weight by another 10

Completed 5k runs twice this week

Nutrition/meal plan review. Any changes to make?

Raise daily protein intake by another 10g

Things to work on and targets for next week:

Complete two weight sessions for shoulders

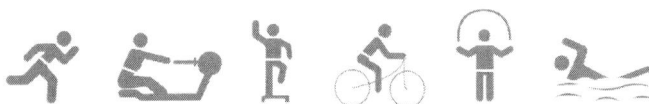

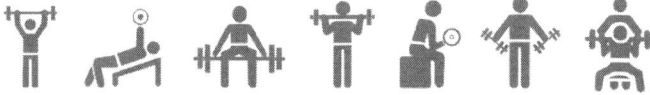

WEEKLY REVIEW

Week of :

EXERCISE	Number of sessions	Mon	Tue	Wed	Thu	Fri	Sat	Sun
Weight Training								
Cardio								
Stretching								

Muscle Group(s)	Number of sessions	Mon	Tue	Wed	Thu	Fri	Sat	Sun
Chest								
Shoulders								
Back								
Arms								
Legs								
Abs								

Weekly training target(s) achieved?					Yes		No	

Did I sleep for 56 hrs in the week?	Mon	Tue	Wed	Thu	Fri	Sat	Sun
Total Sleep Hours							

Notes:

Highlight/achievement of the week:

Nutrition/meal plan review. Any changes to make?

Things to work on and targets for next week:

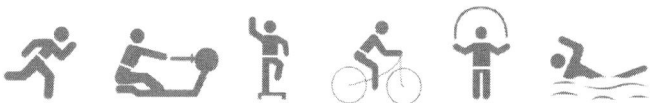

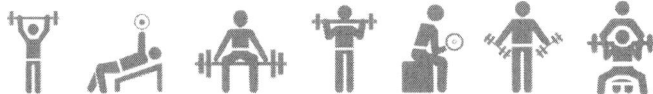

WEEKLY REVIEW   Week of :

EXERCISE	Number of sessions	Mon	Tue	Wed	Thu	Fri	Sat	Sun
Weight Training								
Cardio								
Stretching								

Muscle Group(s)	Number of sessions	Mon	Tue	Wed	Thu	Fri	Sat	Sun
Chest								
Shoulders								
Back								
Arms								
Legs								
Abs								

Weekly training target(s) achieved?				Yes		No	

Did I sleep for 56 hrs in the week?	Mon	Tue	Wed	Thu	Fri	Sat	Sun
Total Sleep Hours							

Notes:

Highlight/achievement of the week:

Nutrition/meal plan review. Any changes to make?

Things to work on and targets for next week:

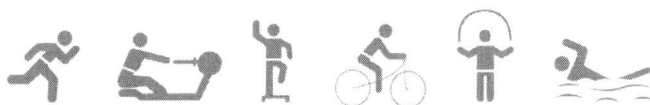

WEEKLY REVIEW   Week of :

EXERCISE	Number of sessions	Mon	Tue	Wed	Thu	Fri	Sat	Sun
Weight Training								
Cardio								
Stretching								

Muscle Group(s)	Number of sessions	Mon	Tue	Wed	Thu	Fri	Sat	Sun
Chest								
Shoulders								
Back								
Arms								
Legs								
Abs								

Weekly training target(s) achieved?				Yes		No	

Did I sleep for 56 hrs in the week?	Mon	Tue	Wed	Thu	Fri	Sat	Sun
Total Sleep Hours							

Notes:

Highlight/achievement of the week:

Nutrition/meal plan review. Any changes to make?

Things to work on and targets for next week:

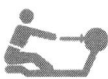 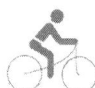

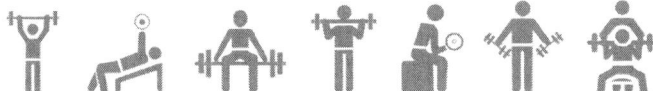

WEEKLY REVIEW   Week of :

EXERCISE	Number of sessions	Mon	Tue	Wed	Thu	Fri	Sat	Sun
Weight Training								
Cardio								
Stretching								

Muscle Group(s)	Number of sessions	Mon	Tue	Wed	Thu	Fri	Sat	Sun
Chest								
Shoulders								
Back								
Arms								
Legs								
Abs								

Weekly training target(s) achieved?		Yes		No	

Did I sleep for 56 hrs in the week?	Mon	Tue	Wed	Thu	Fri	Sat	Sun
Total Sleep Hours							

Notes:

Highlight/achievement of the week:

Nutrition/meal plan review. Any changes to make?

Things to work on and targets for next week:

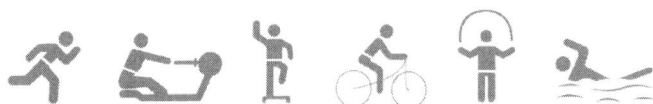

WEEKLY REVIEW   Week of :

EXERCISE	Number of sessions	Mon	Tue	Wed	Thu	Fri	Sat	Sun
Weight Training								
Cardio								
Stretching								

Muscle Group(s)	Number of sessions	Mon	Tue	Wed	Thu	Fri	Sat	Sun
Chest								
Shoulders								
Back								
Arms								
Legs								
Abs								

Weekly training target(s) achieved?				Yes		No	

Did I sleep for 56 hrs in the week?	Mon	Tue	Wed	Thu	Fri	Sat	Sun
Total Sleep Hours							

Notes:

Highlight/achievement of the week:

Nutrition/meal plan review. Any changes to make?

Things to work on and targets for next week:

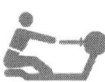
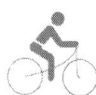

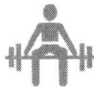

WEEKLY REVIEW   Week of :

EXERCISE	Number of sessions	Mon	Tue	Wed	Thu	Fri	Sat	Sun
Weight Training								
Cardio								
Stretching								
Muscle Group(s)	Number of sessions	Mon	Tue	Wed	Thu	Fri	Sat	Sun
Chest								
Shoulders								
Back								
Arms								
Legs								
Abs								

Weekly training target(s) achieved?				Yes		No	

Did I sleep for 56 hrs in the week?	Mon	Tue	Wed	Thu	Fri	Sat	Sun
Total Sleep Hours							

Notes:

Highlight/achievement of the week:

Nutrition/meal plan review. Any changes to make?

Things to work on and targets for next week:

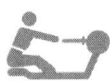 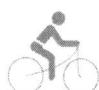 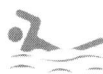

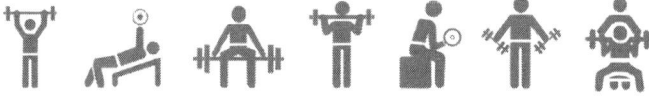

WEEKLY REVIEW   *Week of :*

EXERCISE	*Number of sessions*	Mon	Tue	Wed	Thu	Fri	Sat	Sun
Weight Training								
Cardio								
Stretching								

Muscle Group(s)	*Number of sessions*	Mon	Tue	Wed	Thu	Fri	Sat	Sun
Chest								
Shoulders								
Back								
Arms								
Legs								
Abs								

Weekly training target(s) achieved?					Yes		No	

Did I sleep for 56 hrs in the week?	Mon	Tue	Wed	Thu	Fri	Sat	Sun
Total Sleep Hours							

Notes:

Highlight/achievement of the week:

Nutrition/meal plan review. Any changes to make?

Things to work on and targets for next week:

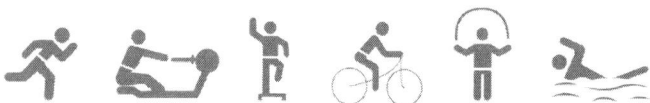

WEEKLY REVIEW   Week of :

EXERCISE	Number of sessions	Mon	Tue	Wed	Thu	Fri	Sat	Sun
Weight Training								
Cardio								
Stretching								

Muscle Group(s)	Number of sessions	Mon	Tue	Wed	Thu	Fri	Sat	Sun
Chest								
Shoulders								
Back								
Arms								
Legs								
Abs								

Weekly training target(s) achieved?				Yes		No	

Did I sleep for 56 hrs in the week?	Mon	Tue	Wed	Thu	Fri	Sat	Sun
Total Sleep Hours							

Notes:

Highlight/achievement of the week:

Nutrition/meal plan review. Any changes to make?

Things to work on and targets for next week:

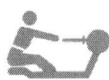
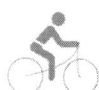

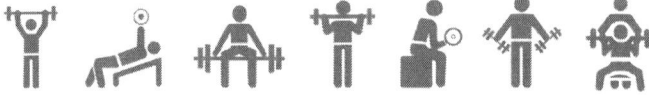

WEEKLY REVIEW

Week of :

EXERCISE	Number of sessions	Mon	Tue	Wed	Thu	Fri	Sat	Sun
Weight Training								
Cardio								
Stretching								

Muscle Group(s)	Number of sessions	Mon	Tue	Wed	Thu	Fri	Sat	Sun
Chest								
Shoulders								
Back								
Arms								
Legs								
Abs								

Weekly training target(s) achieved?				Yes		No	

Did I sleep for 56 hrs in the week?	Mon	Tue	Wed	Thu	Fri	Sat	Sun
Total Sleep Hours							

Notes:

Highlight/achievement of the week:

Nutrition/meal plan review. Any changes to make?

Things to work on and targets for next week:

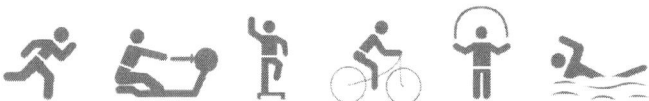

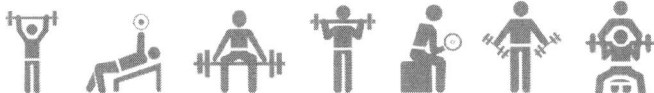

WEEKLY REVIEW   Week of :

EXERCISE	Number of sessions	Mon	Tue	Wed	Thu	Fri	Sat	Sun
Weight Training								
Cardio								
Stretching								

Muscle Group(s)	Number of sessions	Mon	Tue	Wed	Thu	Fri	Sat	Sun
Chest								
Shoulders								
Back								
Arms								
Legs								
Abs								

Weekly training target(s) achieved?					Yes		No	

Did I sleep for 56 hrs in the week?	Mon	Tue	Wed	Thu	Fri	Sat	Sun
Total Sleep Hours							

Notes:

Highlight/achievement of the week:

Nutrition/meal plan review. Any changes to make?

Things to work on and targets for next week:

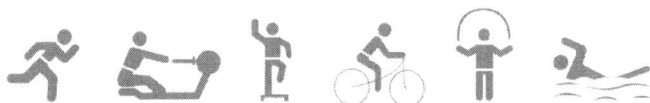

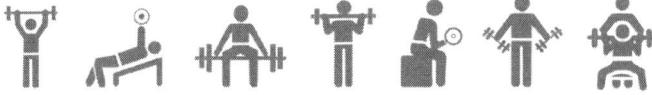

WEEKLY REVIEW   Week of :

EXERCISE	Number of sessions	Mon	Tue	Wed	Thu	Fri	Sat	Sun
Weight Training								
Cardio								
Stretching								

Muscle Group(s)	Number of sessions	Mon	Tue	Wed	Thu	Fri	Sat	Sun
Chest								
Shoulders								
Back								
Arms								
Legs								
Abs								

Weekly training target(s) achieved?					Yes		No	

Did I sleep for 56 hrs in the week?	Mon	Tue	Wed	Thu	Fri	Sat	Sun
Total Sleep Hours							

Notes:

Highlight/achievement of the week:

Nutrition/meal plan review. Any changes to make?

Things to work on and targets for next week:

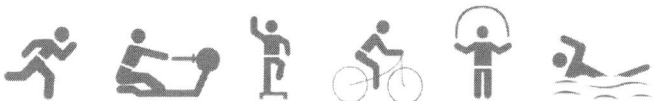

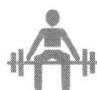

WEEKLY REVIEW   Week of :

EXERCISE	Number of sessions	Mon	Tue	Wed	Thu	Fri	Sat	Sun
Weight Training								
Cardio								
Stretching								
Muscle Group(s)	*Number of sessions*	Mon	Tue	Wed	Thu	Fri	Sat	Sun
Chest								
Shoulders								
Back								
Arms								
Legs								
Abs								

Weekly training target(s) achieved?				Yes		No	

Did I sleep for 56 hrs in the week?	Mon	Tue	Wed	Thu	Fri	Sat	Sun
Total Sleep Hours							

Notes:

Highlight/achievement of the week:

Nutrition/meal plan review. Any changes to make?

Things to work on and targets for next week:

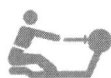 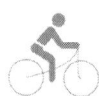

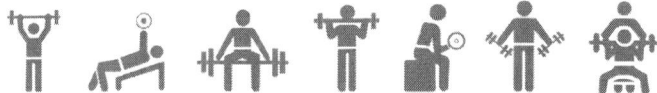

WEEKLY REVIEW   Week of :

EXERCISE	Number of sessions	Mon	Tue	Wed	Thu	Fri	Sat	Sun
Weight Training								
Cardio								
Stretching								

Muscle Group(s)	Number of sessions	Mon	Tue	Wed	Thu	Fri	Sat	Sun
Chest								
Shoulders								
Back								
Arms								
Legs								
Abs								

Weekly training target(s) achieved?					Yes		No	

Did I sleep for 56 hrs in the week?	Mon	Tue	Wed	Thu	Fri	Sat	Sun
Total Sleep Hours							

Notes:

Highlight/achievement of the week:

Nutrition/meal plan review. Any changes to make?

Things to work on and targets for next week:

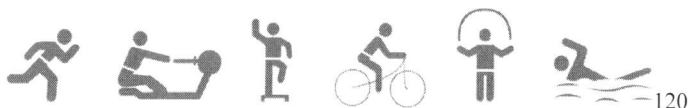

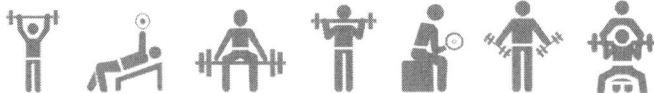

WEEKLY REVIEW

Week of :

EXERCISE	Number of sessions	Mon	Tue	Wed	Thu	Fri	Sat	Sun
Weight Training								
Cardio								
Stretching								

Muscle Group(s)	Number of sessions	Mon	Tue	Wed	Thu	Fri	Sat	Sun
Chest								
Shoulders								
Back								
Arms								
Legs								
Abs								

Weekly training target(s) achieved?					Yes		No	

Did I sleep for 56 hrs in the week?	Mon	Tue	Wed	Thu	Fri	Sat	Sun
Total Sleep Hours							

Notes:

Highlight/achievement of the week:

Nutrition/meal plan review. Any changes to make?

Things to work on and targets for next week:

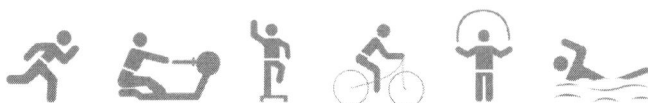

WEEKLY REVIEW   Week of :

EXERCISE	Number of sessions	Mon	Tue	Wed	Thu	Fri	Sat	Sun
Weight Training								
Cardio								
Stretching								

Muscle Group(s)	Number of sessions	Mon	Tue	Wed	Thu	Fri	Sat	Sun
Chest								
Shoulders								
Back								
Arms								
Legs								
Abs								

Weekly training target(s) achieved?					Yes		No	

Did I sleep for 56 hrs in the week?	Mon	Tue	Wed	Thu	Fri	Sat	Sun
Total Sleep Hours							

Notes:

Highlight/achievement of the week:

Nutrition/meal plan review. Any changes to make?

Things to work on and targets for next week:

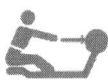 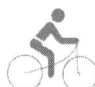

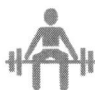

WEEKLY REVIEW   Week of :

EXERCISE	Number of sessions	Mon	Tue	Wed	Thu	Fri	Sat	Sun
Weight Training								
Cardio								
Stretching								

Muscle Group(s)	Number of sessions	Mon	Tue	Wed	Thu	Fri	Sat	Sun
Chest								
Shoulders								
Back								
Arms								
Legs								
Abs								

Weekly training target(s) achieved?						Yes		No

Did I sleep for 56 hrs in the week?	Mon	Tue	Wed	Thu	Fri	Sat	Sun
Total Sleep Hours							

Notes:

Highlight/achievement of the week:

Nutrition/meal plan review. Any changes to make?

Things to work on and targets for next week:

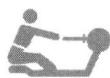 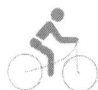

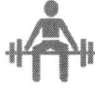

WEEKLY REVIEW   Week of :

EXERCISE	Number of sessions	Mon	Tue	Wed	Thu	Fri	Sat	Sun
Weight Training								
Cardio								
Stretching								
Muscle Group(s)	Number of sessions	Mon	Tue	Wed	Thu	Fri	Sat	Sun
Chest								
Shoulders								
Back								
Arms								
Legs								
Abs								

Weekly training target(s) achieved?					Yes		No	

Did I sleep for 56 hrs in the week?	Mon	Tue	Wed	Thu	Fri	Sat	Sun
Total Sleep Hours							

Notes:

Highlight/achievement of the week:

Nutrition/meal plan review. Any changes to make?

Things to work on and targets for next week:

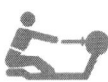 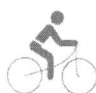

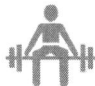

WEEKLY REVIEW   Week of :

EXERCISE	Number of sessions	Mon	Tue	Wed	Thu	Fri	Sat	Sun
Weight Training								
Cardio								
Stretching								

Muscle Group(s)	Number of sessions	Mon	Tue	Wed	Thu	Fri	Sat	Sun
Chest								
Shoulders								
Back								
Arms								
Legs								
Abs								

Weekly training target(s) achieved?				Yes		No	

Did I sleep for 56 hrs in the week?	Mon	Tue	Wed	Thu	Fri	Sat	Sun
Total Sleep Hours							

Notes:

Highlight/achievement of the week:

Nutrition/meal plan review. Any changes to make?

Things to work on and targets for next week:

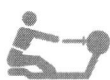
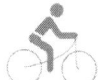

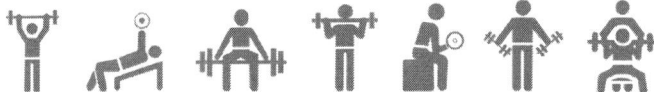

WEEKLY REVIEW   Week of :

EXERCISE	*Number of sessions*	Mon	Tue	Wed	Thu	Fri	Sat	Sun
Weight Training								
Cardio								
Stretching								

Muscle Group(s)	*Number of sessions*	Mon	Tue	Wed	Thu	Fri	Sat	Sun
Chest								
Shoulders								
Back								
Arms								
Legs								
Abs								

Weekly training target(s) achieved?					Yes		No	

Did I sleep for 56 hrs in the week?		Mon	Tue	Wed	Thu	Fri	Sat	Sun
Total Sleep Hours								

Notes:

Highlight/achievement of the week:

Nutrition/meal plan review. Any changes to make?

Things to work on and targets for next week:

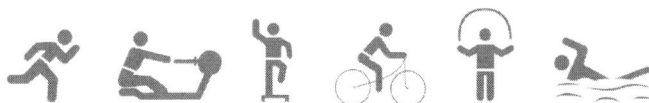

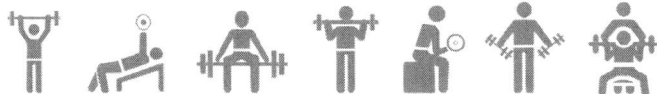

WEEKLY REVIEW   Week of :

EXERCISE	Number of sessions	Mon	Tue	Wed	Thu	Fri	Sat	Sun
Weight Training								
Cardio								
Stretching								

Muscle Group(s)	Number of sessions	Mon	Tue	Wed	Thu	Fri	Sat	Sun
Chest								
Shoulders								
Back								
Arms								
Legs								
Abs								

Weekly training target(s) achieved?					Yes		No	

Did I sleep for 56 hrs in the week?	Mon	Tue	Wed	Thu	Fri	Sat	Sun
Total Sleep Hours							

Notes:

Highlight/achievement of the week:

Nutrition/meal plan review. Any changes to make?

Things to work on and targets for next week:

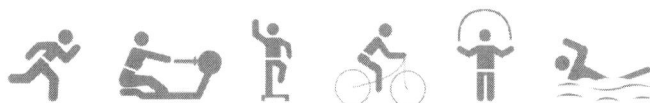

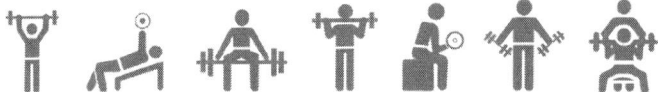

WEEKLY REVIEW   Week of :

EXERCISE	Number of sessions	Mon	Tue	Wed	Thu	Fri	Sat	Sun
Weight Training								
Cardio								
Stretching								

Muscle Group(s)	Number of sessions	Mon	Tue	Wed	Thu	Fri	Sat	Sun
Chest								
Shoulders								
Back								
Arms								
Legs								
Abs								

Weekly training target(s) achieved?					Yes		No	

Did I sleep for 56 hrs in the week?	Mon	Tue	Wed	Thu	Fri	Sat	Sun
Total Sleep Hours							

Notes:

Highlight/achievement of the week:

Nutrition/meal plan review. Any changes to make?

Things to work on and targets for next week:

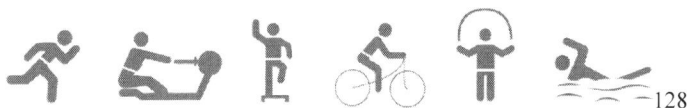

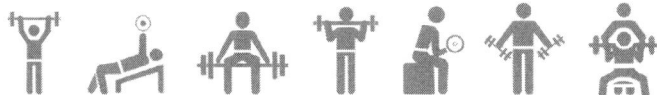

WEEKLY REVIEW   Week of :

EXERCISE	Number of sessions	Mon	Tue	Wed	Thu	Fri	Sat	Sun
Weight Training								
Cardio								
Stretching								

Muscle Group(s)	Number of sessions	Mon	Tue	Wed	Thu	Fri	Sat	Sun
Chest								
Shoulders								
Back								
Arms								
Legs								
Abs								

Weekly training target(s) achieved?					Yes		No	

Did I sleep for 56 hrs in the week?	Mon	Tue	Wed	Thu	Fri	Sat	Sun
Total Sleep Hours							

Notes:

Highlight/achievement of the week:

Nutrition/meal plan review. Any changes to make?

Things to work on and targets for next week:

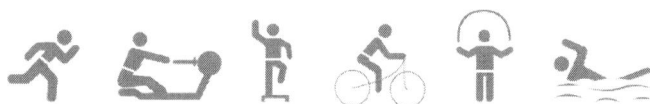

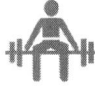

WEEKLY REVIEW   Week of :

EXERCISE	Number of sessions	Mon	Tue	Wed	Thu	Fri	Sat	Sun
Weight Training								
Cardio								
Stretching								

Muscle Group(s)	Number of sessions	Mon	Tue	Wed	Thu	Fri	Sat	Sun
Chest								
Shoulders								
Back								
Arms								
Legs								
Abs								

Weekly training target(s) achieved?					Yes		No	

Did I sleep for 56 hrs in the week?	Mon	Tue	Wed	Thu	Fri	Sat	Sun
Total Sleep Hours							

Notes:

Highlight/achievement of the week:

Nutrition/meal plan review. Any changes to make?

Things to work on and targets for next week:

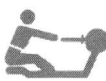
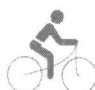

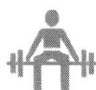

WEEKLY REVIEW

Week of :

EXERCISE	Number of sessions	Mon	Tue	Wed	Thu	Fri	Sat	Sun
Weight Training								
Cardio								
Stretching								

Muscle Group(s)	Number of sessions	Mon	Tue	Wed	Thu	Fri	Sat	Sun
Chest								
Shoulders								
Back								
Arms								
Legs								
Abs								

Weekly training target(s) achieved?					Yes		No	

Did I sleep for 56 hrs in the week?	Mon	Tue	Wed	Thu	Fri	Sat	Sun
Total Sleep Hours							

Notes:

Highlight/achievement of the week:

Nutrition/meal plan review. Any changes to make?

Things to work on and targets for next week:

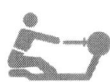 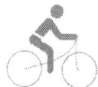 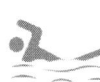

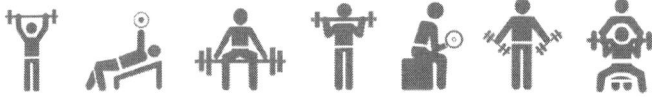

WEEKLY REVIEW

Week of :

EXERCISE	Number of sessions	Mon	Tue	Wed	Thu	Fri	Sat	Sun
Weight Training								
Cardio								
Stretching								

Muscle Group(s)	Number of sessions	Mon	Tue	Wed	Thu	Fri	Sat	Sun
Chest								
Shoulders								
Back								
Arms								
Legs								
Abs								

Weekly training target(s) achieved?						Yes		No	

Did I sleep for 56 hrs in the week?	Mon	Tue	Wed	Thu	Fri	Sat	Sun
Total Sleep Hours							

Notes:

Highlight/achievement of the week:

Nutrition/meal plan review. Any changes to make?

Things to work on and targets for next week:

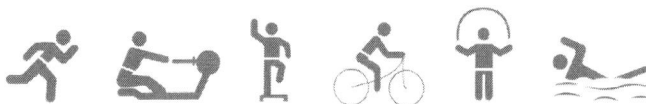

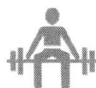

WEEKLY REVIEW   *Week of :*

EXERCISE	Number of sessions	Mon	Tue	Wed	Thu	Fri	Sat	Sun
Weight Training								
Cardio								
Stretching								

Muscle Group(s)	Number of sessions	Mon	Tue	Wed	Thu	Fri	Sat	Sun
Chest								
Shoulders								
Back								
Arms								
Legs								
Abs								

Weekly training target(s) achieved?				Yes		No	

Did I sleep for 56 hrs in the week?	Mon	Tue	Wed	Thu	Fri	Sat	Sun
Total Sleep Hours							

Notes:

Highlight/achievement of the week:

Nutrition/meal plan review. Any changes to make?

Things to work on and targets for next week:

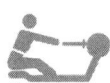 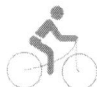

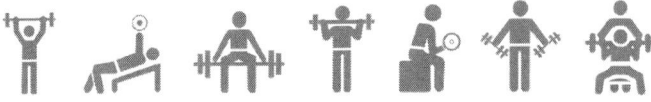

Monthly Progress Review

New month, bigger goals!

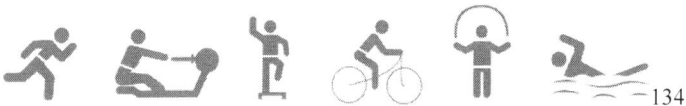

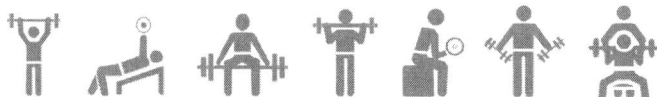

MONTHLY ASSESSMENT　　　Month of : *July 2018*

Body Measurements	Chest	Biceps	Forearms	Waist	Hips	Thighs
Actual	44	16	10	34	38	22
Goal	48	16	14	32	36	25

Body Weight/Fat Actual: *80kg/16%*　　**Body Weight/Fat Goal:** *80kg/17%*

Number of sessions	Week 1	Week 2	Week 3	Week 4	Week 5	Total
WEIGHT TRAINING	4	3	4	4	2	17
CARDIO	3	3	3	2	1	12
STRETCHING	4	4	4	4	2	18
Yoga	1	2	1	1	-	5

Muscle Group sessions	Week 1	Week 2	Week 3	Week 4	Week 5	Total
Chest	2	2	2	1	1	8
Shoulders	1	2	1	2	-	6
Back	2	2	2	1	-	7
Arms	2	2	2	2	1	9
Legs	2	1	2	2	1	8
Abs	3	3	2	3	1	12

Target(s) achieved? Yes/No	Week 1	Week 2	Week 3	Week 4	Week 5	Overall for the Month
Weight Training	✓	✓	✓		✓	✓
Cardio	✓	✓		✓	✓	✓
Sleep Hours	✓		✓		✓	
Meal / Nutrition	✓	✓	✓	✓	✓	✓

Notes

Highlights/achievements of the month:

Reduced my body fat down to 16%

Goal(s) for next month and areas of improvement:

Increase chest measurement to 46, and biceps to 18

Make sure to achieve the sleep hours target

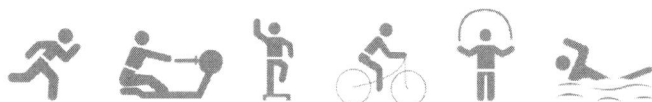

MONTHLY ASSESSMENT   Month of :

Body Measurements	Chest	Biceps	Forearms	Waist	Hips	Thighs
Actual						
Goal						

Body Weight/Fat Actual: **Body Weight/Fat Goal:**

Number of sessions	Week 1	Week 2	Week 3	Week 4	Week 5	Total
WEIGHT TRAINING						
CARDIO						
STRETCHING						

Muscle Group sessions	Week 1	Week 2	Week 3	Week 4	Week 5	Total
Chest						
Shoulders						
Back						
Arms						
Legs						
Abs						

Target(s) achieved? Yes/No	Week 1	Week 2	Week 3	Week 4	Week 5	Overall for the Month
Weight Training						
Cardio						
Sleep Hours						
Meal / Nutrition						
Notes						

Highlights/achievements of the month:

Goal(s) for next month and areas of improvement:

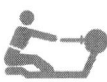 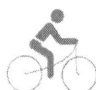

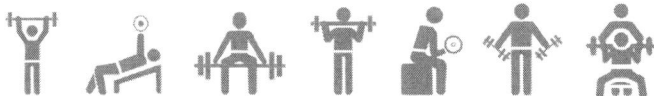

MONTHLY ASSESSMENT   Month of :

Body Measurements	Chest	Biceps	Forearms	Waist	Hips	Thighs
Actual						
Goal						

Body Weight/Fat Actual: **Body Weight/Fat Goal:**

Number of sessions	Week 1	Week 2	Week 3	Week 4	Week 5	Total
WEIGHT TRAINING						
CARDIO						
STRETCHING						

Muscle Group sessions	Week 1	Week 2	Week 3	Week 4	Week 5	Total
Chest						
Shoulders						
Back						
Arms						
Legs						
Abs						

Target(s) achieved? Yes/No	Week 1	Week 2	Week 3	Week 4	Week 5	Overall for the Month
Weight Training						
Cardio						
Sleep Hours						
Meal / Nutrition						
Notes						

Highlights/achievements of the month:

Goal(s) for next month and areas of improvement:

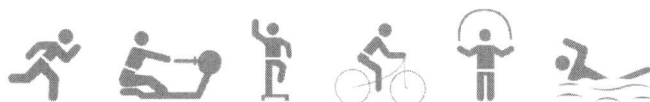

MONTHLY ASSESSMENT   Month of :

Body Measurements	Chest	Biceps	Forearms	Waist	Hips	Thighs
Actual						
Goal						

Body Weight/Fat Actual: **Body Weight/Fat Goal:**

Number of sessions	Week 1	Week 2	Week 3	Week 4	Week 5	Total
WEIGHT TRAINING						
CARDIO						
STRETCHING						

Muscle Group sessions	Week 1	Week 2	Week 3	Week 4	Week 5	Total
Chest						
Shoulders						
Back						
Arms						
Legs						
Abs						

Target(s) achieved? Yes/No	Week 1	Week 2	Week 3	Week 4	Week 5	Overall for the Month
Weight Training						
Cardio						
Sleep Hours						
Meal / Nutrition						

Notes

Highlights/achievements of the month:

Goal(s) for next month and areas of improvement:

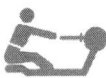
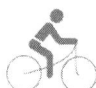

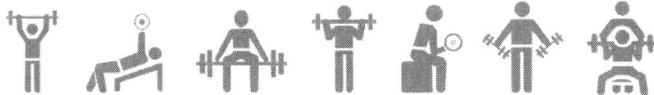

MONTHLY ASSESSMENT   Month of :

Body Measurements	Chest	Biceps	Forearms	Waist	Hips	Thighs
Actual						
Goal						

Body Weight/Fat Actual: **Body Weight/Fat Goal:**

Number of sessions	Week 1	Week 2	Week 3	Week 4	Week 5	Total
WEIGHT TRAINING						
CARDIO						
STRETCHING						

Muscle Group sessions	Week 1	Week 2	Week 3	Week 4	Week 5	Total
Chest						
Shoulders						
Back						
Arms						
Legs						
Abs						

Target(s) achieved? Yes/No	Week 1	Week 2	Week 3	Week 4	Week 5	Overall for the Month
Weight Training						
Cardio						
Sleep Hours						
Meal / Nutrition						
Notes						

Highlights/achievements of the month:

Goal(s) for next month and areas of improvement:

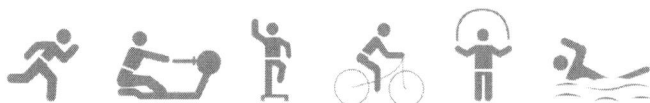

MONTHLY ASSESSMENT   Month of :

Body Measurements	Chest	Biceps	Forearms	Waist	Hips	Thighs
Actual						
Goal						

Body Weight/Fat Actual: **Body Weight/Fat Goal:**

Number of sessions	Week 1	Week 2	Week 3	Week 4	Week 5	Total
WEIGHT TRAINING						
CARDIO						
STRETCHING						

Muscle Group sessions	Week 1	Week 2	Week 3	Week 4	Week 5	Total
Chest						
Shoulders						
Back						
Arms						
Legs						
Abs						

Target(s) achieved? Yes/No	Week 1	Week 2	Week 3	Week 4	Week 5	Overall for the Month
Weight Training						
Cardio						
Sleep Hours						
Meal / Nutrition						

Notes

Highlights/achievements of the month:

Goal(s) for next month and areas of improvement:

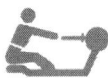
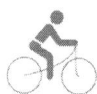
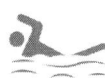

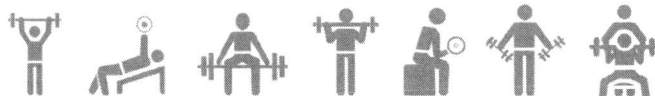

MONTHLY ASSESSMENT   Month of :

Body Measurements	Chest	Biceps	Forearms	Waist	Hips	Thighs
Actual						
Goal						

Body Weight/Fat Actual:			Body Weight/Fat Goal:			

Number of sessions	Week 1	Week 2	Week 3	Week 4	Week 5	Total
WEIGHT TRAINING						
CARDIO						
STRETCHING						

Muscle Group sessions	Week 1	Week 2	Week 3	Week 4	Week 5	Total
Chest						
Shoulders						
Back						
Arms						
Legs						
Abs						

Target(s) achieved? Yes/No	Week 1	Week 2	Week 3	Week 4	Week 5	Overall for the Month
Weight Training						
Cardio						
Sleep Hours						
Meal / Nutrition						
Notes						

Highlights/achievements of the month:

Goal(s) for next month and areas of improvement:

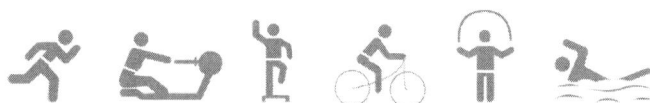

MONTHLY ASSESSMENT   Month of :

Body Measurements	Chest	Biceps	Forearms	Waist	Hips	Thighs
Actual						
Goal						

Body Weight/Fat Actual: **Body Weight/Fat Goal:**

Number of sessions	Week 1	Week 2	Week 3	Week 4	Week 5	Total
WEIGHT TRAINING						
CARDIO						
STRETCHING						

Muscle Group sessions	Week 1	Week 2	Week 3	Week 4	Week 5	Total
Chest						
Shoulders						
Back						
Arms						
Legs						
Abs						

Target(s) achieved? Yes/No	Week 1	Week 2	Week 3	Week 4	Week 5	Overall for the Month
Weight Training						
Cardio						
Sleep Hours						
Meal / Nutrition						

Notes

Highlights/achievements of the month:

Goal(s) for next month and areas of improvement:

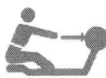

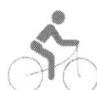

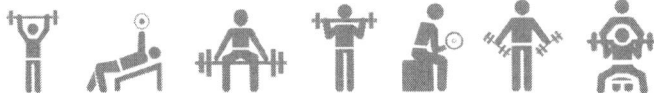

MONTHLY ASSESSMENT   Month of :

Body Measurements	Chest	Biceps	Forearms	Waist	Hips	Thighs
Actual						
Goal						

Body Weight/Fat Actual: **Body Weight/Fat Goal:**

Number of sessions	Week 1	Week 2	Week 3	Week 4	Week 5	Total
WEIGHT TRAINING						
CARDIO						
STRETCHING						

Muscle Group sessions	Week 1	Week 2	Week 3	Week 4	Week 5	Total
Chest						
Shoulders						
Back						
Arms						
Legs						
Abs						

Target(s) achieved? Yes/No	Week 1	Week 2	Week 3	Week 4	Week 5	Overall for the Month
Weight Training						
Cardio						
Sleep Hours						
Meal / Nutrition						
Notes						

Highlights/achievements of the month:

Goal(s) for next month and areas of improvement:

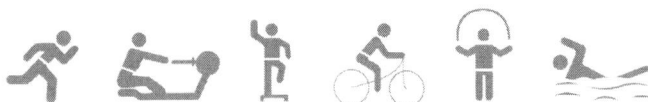

Reference Exercises	
Chest	Flat/incline/decline bench press
	Flat/incline dumbell press
	Dumbell flys
	Dips/push-ups
	Single arm dumbell press
	Cable crossover flys
	Dumbell pullovers
Triceps	Close grip bench press
	Lying overhead extensions
	Kickbacks
	Cable pushdowns
Biceps	Standing dumbell curls
	Incline dumbell hammer curls
	Incline inner biceps curls
	Wide/regular grip barbell curls
Forearms	Hammer curls
	Wrist curls
	Reverse curls
Shoulders	Seated press
	Alternate dumbell press
	Lateral raises
	Front raises
Back	Pull-ups
	Lateral pulldown
	Machine/dumbell rows
	Bent over rows
	Dead-lifts
	Close grip cable pulldowns
	T-bar rows
Legs	Squats
	Dead lifts
	Forward lunges
	Calf raises
	Single leg raises
Abs	Lying crunches
	Dumbell woodchop
	Bentover rows
	Cable crunches

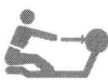

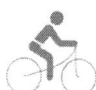

Fitness Goals	Date Planned	Date Achieved

Fitness Goals	Date Planned	Date Achieved

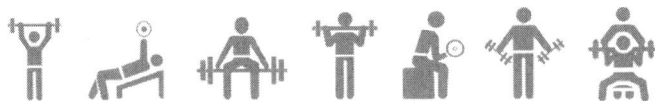

Notes

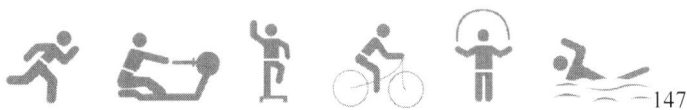

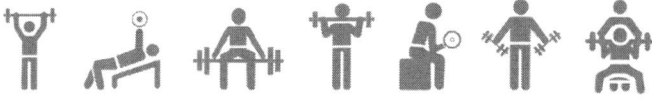

Notes

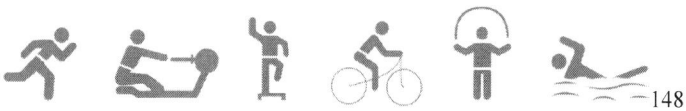

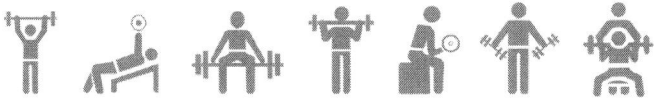

Notes

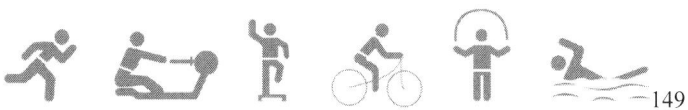

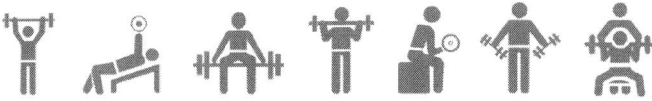

LEGAL NOTES

39143318R10083

Printed in Great Britain
by Amazon